The History of Medicine: A Very Short Introduction

Very Short Introductions available now:

ADVERTISING Winston Fletcher
AFRICAN HISTORY John Parker and Richard Rathbone
AGNOSTICISM Robin Le Poidevin
AMERICAN POLITICAL PARTIES AND ELECTIONS L. Sandy Maisel
THE AMERICAN PRESIDENCY Charles O. Jones
ANARCHISM Colin Ward
ANCIENT EGYPT Ian Shaw
ANCIENT PHILOSOPHY Julia Annas
ANCIENT WARFARE Harry Sidebottom
ANGLICANISM Mark Chapman
THE ANGLO-SAXON AGE John Blair
ANIMAL RIGHTS David DeGrazia
ANTISEMITISM Steven Beller
THE APOCRYPHAL GOSPELS Paul Foster
ARCHAEOLOGY Paul Bahn
ARCHITECTURE Andrew Ballantyne
ARISTOCRACY William Doyle
ARISTOTLE Jonathan Barnes
ART HISTORY Dana Arnold
ART THEORY Cynthia Freeland
ATHEISM Julian Baggini
AUGUSTINE Henry Chadwick
AUTISM Uta Frith
BARTHES Jonathan Culler
BESTSELLERS John Sutherland
THE BIBLE John Riches
BIBLICAL ARCHEOLOGY Eric H. Cline
BIOGRAPHY Hermione Lee
THE BLUES Elijah Wald
THE BOOK OF MORMON Terryl Givens
THE BRAIN Michael O'Shea
BRITISH POLITICS Anthony Wright
BUDDHA Michael Carrithers
BUDDHISM Damien Keown
BUDDHIST ETHICS Damien Keown
CAPITALISM James Fulcher
CATHOLICISM Gerald O'Collins
THE CELTS Barry Cunliffe
CHAOS Leonard Smith
CHOICE THEORY Michael Allingham
CHRISTIAN ART Beth Williamson
CHRISTIAN ETHICS D. Stephen Long
CHRISTIANITY Linda Woodhead
CITIZENSHIP Richard Bellamy
CLASSICAL MYTHOLOGY Helen Morales
CLASSICS Mary Beard and John Henderson
CLAUSEWITZ Michael Howard
THE COLD WAR Robert McMahon
COMMUNISM Leslie Holmes
CONSCIOUSNESS Susan Blackmore
CONTEMPORARY ART Julian Stallabrass
CONTINENTAL PHILOSOPHY Simon Critchley
COSMOLOGY Peter Coles
THE CRUSADES Christopher Tyerman
CRYPTOGRAPHY Fred Piper and Sean Murphy
DADA AND SURREALISM David Hopkins
DARWIN Jonathan Howard
THE DEAD SEA SCROLLS Timothy Lim
DEMOCRACY Bernard Crick
DESCARTES Tom Sorell
DESERTS Nick Middleton
DESIGN John Heskett
DINOSAURS David Norman
DIPLOMACY Joseph M. Siracusa
DOCUMENTARY FILM Patricia Aufderheide
DREAMING J. Allan Hobson
DRUGS Leslie Iversen
DRUIDS Barry Cunliffe
THE EARTH Martin Redfern
ECONOMICS Partha Dasgupta
EGYPTIAN MYTH Geraldine Pinch
EIGHTEENTH-CENTURY BRITAIN Paul Langford
THE ELEMENTS Philip Ball
EMOTION Dylan Evans
EMPIRE Stephen Howe
ENGELS Terrell Carver
ENGLISH LITERATURE Jonathan Bate
EPIDEMIOLOGY Roldolfo Saracci
ETHICS Simon Blackburn
THE EUROPEAN John Pinder and Simon Usherwood
EVOLUTION Brian and Deborah Charlesworth
EXISTENTIALISM Thomas Flynn
FASCISM Kevin Passmore
FASHION Rebecca Arnold
FEMINISM Margaret Walters
FILM MUSIC Kathryn Kalinak
THE FIRST WORLD WAR Michael Howard
FORENSIC PSYCHOLOGY David Canter
FORENSIC SCIENCE Jim Fraser

FOSSILS Keith Thomson
FOUCAULT Gary Gutting
FREE SPEECH Nigel Warburton
FREE WILL Thomas Pink
FRENCH LITERATURE John D. Lyons
THE FRENCH REVOLUTION William Doyle
FREUD Anthony Storr
FUNDAMENTALISM Malise Ruthven
GALAXIES John Gribbin
GALILEO Stillman Drake
GAME THEORY Ken Binmore
GANDHI Bhikhu Parekh
GEOGRAPHY John Matthews and David Herbert
GEOPOLITICS Klaus Dodds
GERMAN LITERATURE Nicholas Boyle
GERMAN PHILOSOPHY Andrew Bowie
GLOBAL CATASTROPHES Bill McGuire
GLOBAL WARMING Mark Maslin
GLOBALIZATION Manfred Steger
THE GREAT DEPRESSION AND THE NEW DEAL Eric Rauchway
HABERMAS James Gordon Finlayson
HEGEL Peter Singer
HEIDEGGER Michael Inwood
HIEROGLYPHS Penelope Wilson
HINDUISM Kim Knott
HISTORY John H. Arnold
THE HISTORY OF ASTRONOMY Michael Hoskin
THE HISTORY OF LIFE Michael Benton
THE HISTORY OF MEDICINE William Bynum
THE HISTORY OF TIME Leofranc Holford-Strevens
HIV/AIDS Alan Whiteside
HOBBES RICHARD TUCKHUMAN EVOLUTION Bernard Wood
HUMANISM Stephen Law
HUMAN RIGHTS Andrew Clapham
HUME A. J. Ayer
IDEOLOGY Michael Freeden
INDIAN PHILOSOPHY Sue Hamilton
INFORMATION Luciano Floridi
INNOVATION Mark Dodgson and David Gann
INTELLIGENCE Ian J. Deary
INTERNATIONAL MIGRATION Khalid Koser
INTERNATIONAL RELATIONS Paul Wilkinson
ISLAM Malise Ruthven
ISLAMIC HISTORY Adam Silverstein
JOURNALISM Ian Hargreaves
JUDAISM Norman Solomon
JUNG Anthony Stevens
KABBALAH Joseph Dan
KAFKA Ritchie Robertson
KANT Roger Scruton
KEYNES Robert Skidelsky
KIERKEGAARD Patrick Gardiner
THE KORAN Michael Cook
LANDSCAPES AND GEOMORPHOLOGY Andrew Goudie and Heather Viles
LATE ANTIQUITY Gillian Clark
LAW Raymond Wacks
THE LAWS OF THERMODYNAMICS Peter Atkins
LEADERSHIP Keith Grint
LINCOLN Allen C. Guelzo
LINGUISTICS Peter Matthews
LITERARY THEORY Jonathan Culler
LOCKE John Dunn
LOGIC Graham Priest
MACHIAVELLI Quentin Skinner
THE MARQUIS DE SADE John Phillips
MARX Peter Singer
MARTIN LUTHER Scott H. Hendrix
MATHEMATICS Timothy Gowers
THE MEANING OF LIFE Terry Eagleton
MEDICAL ETHICS Tony Hope
MEDIEVAL BRITAIN John Gillingham and Ralph A. Griffiths
MEMORY JONATHAN K. Foster
MICHAEL FARADAY Frank A. J. L. James
MODERN ART David Cottington
MODERN CHINA Rana Mitter
MODERN IRELAND Senia Pašeta
MODERN JAPAN Christopher Goto-Jones
MODERNISM Christopher Butler
MOLECULES Philip Ball
MORMONISM Richard Lyman Bushman
MUHAMMAD Jonathan A. Brown
MUSIC Nicholas Cook
MYTH Robert A. Segal
NATIONALISM Steven Grosby
NELSON MANDELA Elleke Boehmer
NEOLIBERALISM Manfred Steger and Ravi Roy
THE NEW TESTAMENT Luke Timothy Johnson
THE NEW TESTAMENT AS LITERATURE Kyle Keefer

NEWTON Robert Iliffe
NIETZSCHE Michael Tanner
NINETEENTH-CENTURY BRITAIN Christopher Harvie and H. C. G. Matthew
THE NORMAN CONQUEST George Garnett
NORTH AMERICAN INDIANS Theda Perdue and Michael D. Green
NORTHERN IRELAND Marc Mulholland
NOTHING Frank Close
NUCLEAR WEAPONS Joseph M. Siracusa
THE OLD TESTAMENT Michael D. Coogan
PARTICLE PHYSICS Frank Close
PAUL E. P. Sanders
PENTECOSTALISM William K. Kay
PHILOSOPHY Edward Craig
PHILOSOPHY OF LAW Raymond Wacks
PHILOSOPHY OF SCIENCE Samir Okasha
PHOTOGRAPHY Steve Edwards
PLANETS David A. Rothery
PLATO Julia Annas
POLITICAL PHILOSOPHY David Miller
POLITICS Kenneth Minogue
POSTCOLONIALISM Robert Young
POSTMODERNISM Christopher Butler
POSTSTRUCTURALISM Catherine Belsey
PREHISTORY Chris Gosden
PRESOCRATIC PHILOSOPHY Catherine Osborne
PRIVACY Raymond Wacks
PROGRESSIVISM Walter Nugent
PSYCHIATRY Tom Burns
PSYCHOLOGY Gillian Butler and Freda McManus
PURITANISM Francis J. Bremer
THE QUAKERS Pink Dandelion
QUANTUM THEORY John Polkinghorne
RACISM Ali Rattansi
THE REAGAN REVOLUTION Gil Troy
THE REFORMATION Peter Marshall
RELATIVITY Russell Stannard
RELIGION IN AMERICA Timothy Beal
THE RENAISSANCE Jerry Brotton
RENAISSANCE ART Geraldine A. Johnson
RISK Baruch Fischhoff and John Kadvany
ROMAN BRITAIN Peter Salway
THE ROMAN EMPIRE Christopher Kelly
ROMANTICISM Michael Ferber
ROUSSEAU Robert Wokler
RUSSELL A. C. Grayling
RUSSIAN LITERATURE Catriona Kelly
THE RUSSIAN REVOLUTION S. A. Smith
SCHIZOPHRENIA Chris Frith and Eve Johnstone
SCHOPENHAUER Christopher Janaway
SCIENCE AND RELIGION Thomas Dixon
SCOTLAND Rab Houston
SEXUALITY Véronique Mottier
SHAKESPEARE Germaine Greer
SOCIAL AND CULTURAL ANTHROPOLOGY John Monaghan and Peter Just
SOCIALISM Michael Newman
SOCIOLOGY Steve Bruce
SOCRATES C. C. W. Taylor
THE SOVIET UNION Stephen Lovell
THE SPANISH CIVIL WAR Helen Graham
SPANISH LITERATURE Jo Labanyi
SPINOZA Roger Scruton
STATISTICS David J. Hand
STUART BRITAIN John Morrill
SUPERCONDUCTIVITY Stephen Blundell
TERRORISM Charles Townshend
THEOLOGY David F. Ford
THOMAS AQUINAS Fergus Kerr
TOCQUEVILLE Harvey C. Mansfield
TRAGEDY Adrian Poole
THE TUDORS John Guy
TWENTIETH-CENTURY BRITAIN Kenneth O. Morgan
THE UNITED NATIONS Jussi M. Hanhimäki
THE U.S. CONGRESS Donald A. Ritchie
UTOPIANISM Lyman Tower Sargent
THE VIKINGS Julian Richards
WITCHCRAFT Malcolm Gaskill
WITTGENSTEIN A. C. Grayling
WORLD MUSIC Philip Bohlman
THE WORLD TRADE ORGANIZATION Amrita Narlikar
WRITING AND SCRIPT Andrew Robinson

For more information visit our web site:
www.oup.co.uk/general/vsi/

William Bynum

THE HISTORY OF MEDICINE

A Very Short Introduction

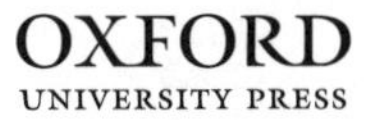

OXFORD
UNIVERSITY PRESS

Great Clarendon Street, Oxford OX2 6DP

Oxford University Press is a department of the University of Oxford.
It furthers the University's objective of excellence in research, scholarship,
and education by publishing worldwide in

Oxford New York

Auckland Cape Town Dar es Salaam Hong Kong Karachi
Kuala Lumpur Madrid Melbourne Mexico City Nairobi
New Delhi Shanghai Taipei Toronto

With offices in

Argentina Austria Brazil Chile Czech Republic France Greece
Guatemala Hungary Italy Japan Poland Portugal Singapore
South Korea Switzerland Thailand Turkey Ukraine Vietnam

Oxford is a registered trade mark of Oxford University Press
in the UK and in certain other countries

Published in the United States
by Oxford University Press Inc., New York

First Published 2008

British Library Cataloguing in Publication Data
Data available

Library of Congress Cataloging in Publication Data
Data available

ISBN 978-0-19-921543-0

7 9 10 8

Typeset by SPI Publisher Services, Pondicherry, India
Printed in Great Britain by
Ashford Colour Press Ltd, Gosport, Hampshire

For Helen

Sine qua non

Contents

Acknowledgements

I have given a short lecture based on the structure of this book to many groups of students. The feedback has been valuable in helping me sort out the forest from the trees.

The staff at Oxford University Press have handled this book with admirable efficiency. The comments of Andrea Keegan and an anonymous referee have improved the style and content. James Thompson has been a model editor. My thanks to them all.

My greatest debt is always to Helen Bynum, who has read the manuscript with wonderful care and expertise. Many years ago, she even heard me give the lecture of the book. She knows how much of this book is hers.

List of illustrations

The publisher and the author apologize for any errors or omissions in the above list. If contacted they will be pleased to rectify these at the earliest opportunity.

Introduction: the kinds of medicine

This is a short book on a very big subject. I have tried to provide a general framework for understanding the history of medicine since the ancient Greeks established what can be called the Western medical tradition. I present my history through a typology of the 'kinds' of medicine. These are summarized in the following table, and expounded in the first five chapters.

The five kinds of medicine in Figure 1 – bedside, library, hospital, community, and laboratory – represent different goals of doctors, as well as reflecting the differing sites in which they work. Although their appearance allows a roughly chronological narrative, these kinds of medicine are cumulative. Bedside medicine, beginning with the Hippocratics, still has resonances in modern primary care, and the library medicine of the Middle Ages is relevant to the information explosion that characterizes the modern medical world (and not, of course, simply the medical one). In the 19th century, hospital medicine was in one sense bedside medicine writ large, with new diagnostic and therapeutic tools, and the medical expertise we expect from the modern hospital. Medicine in the community encompasses the environmental infrastructure of clean water, waste disposal, vaccination programmes, health and safety in our chosen workplaces, along with the analysis of disease patterns and their relationships to diet, habits, or exposure to agents in the

		CHARACTERISTICS			
		OBJECT of INQUIRY	FORM and SITE of EDUCATION	GOAL	EXAMPLE
KINDS	**BEDSIDE**	Whole patient	Apprenticeship	Therapy	Hippocrates (c. 460–370 BCE)
	LIBRARY	Text	Scholastic, linguistic, university	Preservation, recovery, commentary	Constantine the African (d. before 1098)
	HOSPITAL	Patient, organ	Hospital	Diagnosis	R. T. H. Laennec (1781–1826)
	SOCIAL	Population, statistic	Community	Prevent	John Simon (1816–1904)
	LABORATORY	Animal model	Laboratory	Understand	Claude Bernard (1813–1878)

1. The kinds of medicine. A schematic representation of the different 'kinds' of medicine, highlighting the various units of analysis, workplace, and aims that doctors may have. The first five chapters of this book examine these kinds of medicine in their historical contexts

environment. Laboratory medicine takes place mostly in the laboratory, and may be translated into better drugs, and understanding of bodily mechanisms that can improve diagnosis or treatment.

These historical categories are thus still vibrant ones, and they allow a way of thinking about medical history that still resonates with today's citizens who are also taxpayers, consumers of healthcare, and beneficiaries of public health strategies. These 'kinds' of medicine provide both the broad headings for contemporary health budgets, and, especially within the American scene, where special-interest advocacy influences health spending, the identity of interest groups. Primary care, hospital services, public health, biomedical research, and information creation and provision: among major health demands, there is not much else that a modern health minister need bother about. The trouble of course is that these categories in some sense compete with each other, since health budgets are always limited. The more you spend on research, the less you may have for hospital staffing or public health, and vice versa.

The categories overlap historically. In their own ways, the ancient Greeks and Romans developed the whole range of approaches to health-related problems: they tried to prevent diseases within the community, had simple institutions to care for slaves and soldiers, needed places where medical texts were gathered together, tried to add to medical knowledge through enquiry, and of course, cared for patients at the bedside. But the modern categories of hospital, community, and laboratory medicine emerged in their current forms within the 19th century, and are what we think of as 'modernity'. In the final chapter, I use the typology to frame a brief account of major developments in the 20th and 21st centuries, when the 'kinds' of medicine have become intertwined.

The way I have structured this short account privileges the Western medical tradition, which dominates health consumption and expenditure in the West, and is a major force everywhere. There are many other ways in which historians have constructed the story, but I have chosen this one because I believe it has a historically coherent form and is useful in introducing the subject to curious readers.

Were I submitting this manuscript to a medical journal, I would be required to state any competing interests which might colour how I have interpreted my data. I have been a medical historian for almost four decades, but I also trained in medicine, during the 'golden age' that is identified in Chapter 6. My medical education has certainly influenced the way I interpret medicine's past, but I have tried here to avoid either the old-fashioned 'Whiggism', which viewed all history as progress and a series of steps leading inevitably to the present, or the newer version, which has substituted contemporary moral values for intellectual ones and thereby castigates the sexism, racism, and other -isms of our forebears. It seems to me that those in the past who had access have generally sought the medical care that was on offer, and believed that there were good doctors and bad doctors. They wanted a good doctor to take care of them. So do we. What has changed is what constitutes a 'good' doctor.

Chapter 1
Medicine at the bedside

Hippocrates and all that

Hippocrates has become the favoured Father for healers of all stripes. Homoeopathists find in the Hippocratic writings the roots of their doctrines. Naturopaths, chiropractors, herbalists, and osteopaths invoke him as the founder of the ideals that underlie their own approaches to health, disease, and healing. So do modern hospital consultants, many of whom would have repeated his Oath, or a version of it, when they took their medical degrees.

The reasons for this curious state of affairs can be found in history. For one thing, the historical Hippocrates is sufficiently shadowy to allow a multiplicity of interpretations to be hung from him. He is shadowy but real. He lived on the island of Cos, off the coast of present-day Turkey, from about 460 BCE to 370 BCE. This makes him a bit older than Plato, Aristotle, and the other cosmopolitan creators of classical Greek culture, centred in Athens. His antiquity makes the survival of so many 'Hippocratic' works that much more remarkable; people save what they particularly value.

Besides where and approximately when he lived, we know only a little more. He practised medicine, took pupils for a fee, and had a son. He also achieved a fair degree of fame, since Plato mentioned him. Whether he actually wrote any of the works attributed to him is less clear. He certainly did not write them all, for they were composed over about two centuries by various unknown hands. This means that the Hippocratic Corpus, the 60 or so works and fragments that survive, contain much inconsistency and many points of view. These 'Hippocratic' writings cover many aspects of medicine and surgery, as well as diagnostics, therapeutics, and disease prevention. The Hippocratics offered advice on diet and other aspects of healthy living, and there is a particularly influential treatise on the role of the environment in health and disease. There were thus many 'Hippocratic' stances, and our 'Hippocratic medicine' is a historical construct, achieved by picking out certain themes and theories, and putting them together in a framework that was unknown during the centuries of the composition of the treatises.

Amidst this multiplicity, however, there is one strand that runs through the whole corpus, and makes Hippocrates so attractive to so many modern healers. Hippocratic medicine is holistic. The Hippocratic approach is always to the whole patient and the modern yearning for a holistic medicine finds a natural resting place there. Despite its admirable, positive characteristics, this holism was also rooted in cultural values widespread in Greek society. The ancient Greeks disliked dissection of human bodies. They performed no autopsies to determine the cause of death, and Greek doctors taught no deep anatomy to their apprentices. There were no medical schools in the modern sense of the term. Students learned through their masters, and what they knew was surface anatomy and a shrewd sense of looking carefully at their patients for signs suggesting the likely course of the disease, that is its prognosis, and, especially, whether the patient was likely to recover or not. That there were no hospitals meant that the bedside of this chapter's title was literally the patient's, in his or her own home.

These structures of ancient Greek medicine make it the prototype of modern primary care. The Hippocratic doctor needed to know his patient thoroughly: what his social, economic, and familial circumstances were, how he lived, what he usually ate and drank, whether he had travelled or not, whether he was a slave or free, and what his tendencies to disease were. The theoretical reasons for this were embedded in the Hippocratic writings, of which more below.

If the holism attracts modern complementary healers to the Greek, there are other attributes to Hippocratic medicine that resonate within contemporary scientific medicine. The most important of these is its underlying naturalism. The medical systems of the ancient Near East – Egypt, Syria, Mesopotamia, Babylonia – combine theology and healing. The priest-physician is a common trope. Disease was widely assumed to be the result of divine displeasure, transgressions of various kinds, or magical forces. Diagnosis might involve prayer, interpreting animal entrails, or determining how the patient had transgressed. This mix of magico-religious medicine was also part of the Greek landscape during the Hippocratic period. Healing temples dedicated to the Greek god of medicine, Asclepius, were dotted all over the Greek sphere of influence, including, ironically, a famous one in Hippocrates' own backyard, Cos itself. The most substantial one was on the mainland, at Epidaurus, the extensive remains of which are still extant. These temples were in the hands of resident priests who received patients and interpreted illness on the basis of dreams that patients reported to them. The dreams were probably affected by the presence of holy snakes, which undoubtedly disturbed sleep patterns. By sloughing its skin, the snake was an example of renewal, and a prominent part of the caduceus, symbol of the Greek god of healing (see Figure 4). Curiously, Asclepius and the caduceus, both redolent of magic and religion, have been naturalized as an emblem of modern medicine.

These healing temples were an important part of Greek medical care but the values they embodied had little impact on the

Hippocratic Corpus. The treatises that form it assume that disease has a natural cause, but only once does a Hippocratic author explicitly attack supernatural explanations of disease. This occurs at the beginning of a treatise on epilepsy, called 'The Sacred Disease' in common Greek parlance. It was deemed sacred because epileptic attacks were dramatic, causing as they do a loss of consciousness, foaming at the mouth, relaxation of muscle, bladder, and sphincter control, but also included psychological symptoms which sufferers could sometimes turn to their advantage. Alexander the Great and (later) Julius Caesar were powerful epileptics in antiquity. The opening sentences of 'The Sacred Disease' have been interpreted as a clarion call for a complete naturalism within medicine. They are still compelling, written as they were more than two millennia ago:

> It is thus with regard to the disease called Sacred: it appears to me to be nowise more divine nor more sacred than other diseases, but has a natural cause from which it originates like other affections. Men regard its nature and cause as divine from ignorance and wonder, because it is not at all like to other diseases. And this notion of divinity is kept up by their inability to comprehend it, and the simplicity of the mode by which it is cured, for men are freed from it by purifications and incantations. But if it is reckoned divine because it is wonderful, instead of one there are many diseases which would be sacred.

It is significant that the stance is not irreligious ('nowise more divine nor more sacred than other diseases'), but couched within a framework that could offer an explanation within naturalist terms of the origins of this so-called sacred disease. The Hippocratic author goes on to offer such an explanation: epilepsy is caused by blockage within the brain, so that the regular expulsion of phlegm is stopped, thereby producing malfunctioning of the brain, and the dramatic symptoms of the epileptic seizure. Two further implications are worth noting.

First, this Hippocratic author located consciousness and other mental functions to the brain.

> And men ought to know that from nothing else but the brain come joys, delights, laughter and sports, and sorrows, griefs, despondency, and lamentations. And by this, in an especial manner, we acquire wisdom and knowledge, and see and hear, and know what are foul and what are fair, what are bad and what are good, what are sweet, and what unsavoury; some we discriminate by habit, and some we perceive by their utility.

The centrality of the brain is of course now a commonplace in scientific thinking, but it was not so with the Greeks. Plato followed Hippocrates in viewing the brain as the seat of psychological activity, but Plato's pupil Aristotle believed that the heart is the centre of emotion and other mental functions. After all, when we are anxious or in love, it is in the breast, or heart, not the brain, that we experience such events. The heart, not the brain, beats faster when we are most alive. Besides, Aristotle, an experienced student of embryological development, noted that the first sign of life in the developing chick embryo was the motion within the primitive heart. Almost two millennia later, Shakespeare was to recall this old debate:

> Tell me where is fancy bred.
> Or in the heart or in the head?

Despite our language, which still attributes much to the 'heart', Hippocrates and Plato won that debate.

The second significant point to tease out of this treatise relates to the Hippocratic cause of epilepsy: blocked phlegm. Phlegm might seem the sign of a common cold to us, but it was for the Hippocratics one of four humours, which were constitutive of health and disease, and thus at the heart of Hippocratic physiology and pathology. Although humoral doctrine was not contained in all of the Hippocratic treatises, it can be pieced together and was interpreted by the other giant of ancient Greek medicine, Galen (AD 129–c. 210), as central to medical theory. Galen gave humoral medicine such prestige that it dominated medical thinking until the 18th century.

Humours: the complete system

The four humours were blood, yellow bile, black bile, and phlegm, and as can be seen from the schematic diagram in Figure 2, they constituted a formidable framework for understanding health and disease, and much else besides. They eventually embodied a theory of temperaments, which provided a guide to human personality and susceptibility to disease. The properties of the humours – heat, cold, dryness, moistness – offered a parallel reading of the course of diseases, and of the stages of the individual life cycle. Each of the humours was also linked to one of the four elements – air, fire, earth, water – which Greek natural philosophy

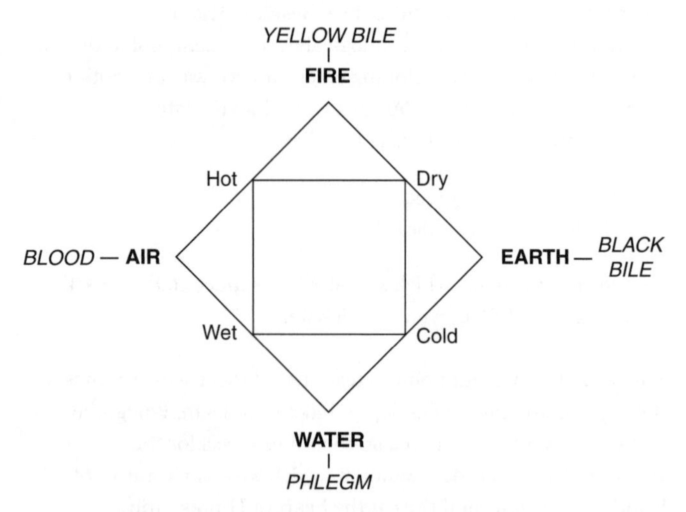

2. The humours: the wonderful simplicity of the Hippocratic scheme is easily recognized, with the equally important qualities (heat, cold, dryness, moistness) which the humours possessed

posited as the constituents of all the things in the sublunary world. Below the moon, in our world, things change, grow old, and die. Above the moon, perfect circular motion was postulated as the norm, with stars made of a fifth element, the 'quintessence'.

Taken as a whole package, Greek humoralism was the most powerful explanatory framework of health and disease available to doctors and laymen until scientific medicine began gradually to replace it during the 19th century.

Bodily fluids and their effects are features that someone caring for a sick person notices. The skin becomes flushed when the sick person is febrile; people cough up phlegm or blood; eyes water and noses run; the urine turns dark if there is jaundice or dehydration; the skin can become clammy, sweaty, or pale; and diarrhoea or vomiting may be prominent features of illness. Greek cultural prohibitions against dissecting human bodies meant that the Hippocratics had relatively little knowledge of deep anatomy, or it was inferred from animal dissections or knowledge acquired through preparation of animals for eating. This did not seem to bother the Hippocratics very much, although Galen later tried very hard to provide anatomical knowledge, largely through dissecting animals.

Humoral medicine does not require all that much knowledge of anatomy, since the operative elements are the bodily fluids, not the solids. Each of the humours was identified with a bodily organ, however: phlegm with the brain, blood with the heart, yellow bile with the liver, and black bile with the spleen. Further, in the surgical treatises of the Hippocratic writings, these doctors also discussed the setting of fractures, reduction of dislocated joints, wound treatment, and simple operations for various specific conditions. Surgical work, then as now, requires a much more focused orientation on a particular area of the body. But Hippocratic *medicine* remained holistic and preoccupied with interpreting the changes of the humours.

Humoralism brought with it two related and enduring themes within Western medicine: balance and moderation. The Hippocratics viewed health as the result of a sound balance of the humours. Imbalance, too much or too little of one or more of them, or an imperfect quality (often described as a corruption) of one of them produced disease. The body was sometimes regarded as a kind of oven, with cooking metaphors prominent in Hippocratic descriptions of disease. Excretions in disease – pus, sweat, expectorated phlegm, concentrated urine, vomitus, diarrhoea – were interpreted as the products of natural defence mechanisms. The body often cooked, or concocted, corrupt or excess humours, to enable the better removal of the surfeit or the peccant humours, and restore a balance.

The Hippocratics interpreted this bedside observation – of the body getting rid of humours – as evidence of what they called the *vix medicatrix naturae*, the healing power of nature. This doctrine has long been debated within medicine, and it was codified in the 19th century with the concept of 'self-limited disease'. A powerful modern medicine is able easily to accommodate it: most disease, treated or untreated, is self-limited. Treating the symptoms of a cold, for example, may make one feel better, but it never really touches the cause, which in due course the body generally deals with. Every doctor knows this, but they also know that the prescription that makes the patient feel better is often interpreted as curative. *Post hoc, ergo propter hoc*: 'after, therefore, because of': a lot of clinical medicine has always relied on this logical fallacy.

The Hippocratics were more modest, and the doctrine of the healing power of nature gave rise to two of their most important aphorisms: 'Natural forces are the healers of disease', and 'As to diseases, make a habit of two things – to help, or at least do no harm'. Therapy was thus aimed primarily at assisting the patient's body do its 'natural' work. Some of their procedures jar with modern sentiment. Bloodletting, for example, had a rational basis, since local inflammation, or the flush of fever, was easily interpreted as evidence that the body had too much blood, and therefore needed aid in ridding itself of it. Bloodletting is one of the oldest and most persistent therapies, and the one most often held up as evidence of the crude barbarity of medicine until the modern period. It continued to be a mainstay of therapeutics until the mid-19th century, and was abandoned only gradually and reluctantly by rank and file practitioners. Patients often demanded it, and many of them reported being helped by having blood let, sometimes so much that the doctor stopped only when the patient was on the point of fainting. As another Hippocratic aphorism put it, 'For extreme diseases, extreme strictness of treatment is most efficacious', often made more pungent: 'Dangerous diseases require dangerous remedies'.

In general, however, humoral therapy was mixed, and included diet, exercise, massage, and other modalities that were aimed at the individual needs of the individual patient. It was this holistic individualism that was the core feature of their medical practice. Although Hippocratic writings contain descriptions of many diseases to which we can give modern labels, they never separated the disease from the individual sufferer. Thus, although we can find accounts of diseases we might call consumption (tuberculosis), stroke, malaria, epilepsy, hysteria, and dysentery, these are presented as events that happened to individual people. They used these experiences to come to generalizations about how to deal with these diseases, presented as aphorisms and what we would now call 'clinical pearls'. Their humoral explanatory framework always encouraged them to tailor particular treatments to unique cases.

The Hippocratics were also acutely aware that diseases often sweep through a community, affecting the old and young, rich and poor, thin and corpulent, male and female: just those attributes that at the bedside they strove to take into account when making a diagnosis and recommending a therapeutic regimen. In two particularly influential treatises, a series of books on *Epidemics*, and one entitled *Airs, Waters, Places*, the Hippocratic writers offered reflections about these wider aspects of disease. *Airs, Waters, Places* is essentially the foundation statement of Western environmentalism, especially as it relates to health and disease. It offered advice on where to build one's house (well-drained soil, protected from chilling winds), and analysed the health of communities in terms of the environmental factors that impinged on their inhabitants. Like most medical and biological thinking until the late 19th century, it espoused what is now called (anachronistically) 'Lamarckianism'; that is, the Hippocratics believed that environmental factors could change the basic characteristics of human beings (skin colour, body shape, and so on), and that these changes could be passed on to offspring. This is an optimistic philosophy of human malleability, consonant with the general Hippocratic confidence that their therapeutic regimen had much to offer to its patients. At the same time, their writings are full of occasions when experience taught that the disease was so far advanced or serious that there was little to be done.

Wider Hippocratic reverberations

The humours provided a theoretical framework that lasted. We still use the idea of the temperaments in casual speech ('a naturally sanguine person', 'generally melancholic'), and the hot–cold, wet–dry axes of the humours regulate how we see common acute complaints. Popular belief has it that we catch colds by going out without our hats on, or getting our feet wet. Doctors, who ought to know better, fall in with popular disease conceptions about the nature and treatment of colds, partly because that is what patients expect, partly because it saves time in the patient–doctor encounter, partly because doctors, too, are all too human. More recently, Darwinian medicine has used the Hippocratic *vix medicatrix naturae* to question the treatment of symptoms. Is it better to suppress the cough, or dry up the nasal secretions, when they are part of a naturally evolved defence?

Much of the Hippocratic legacy was actually transmitted to the West through the writings of Galen, who dominated medical thinking for more than a millennium. Galen saw himself as extending and completing the framework of the Hippocratics. We know much more about him than any other doctor of antiquity: more words of his survive than any other ancient writer, medical or otherwise, and his works are laced with autobiographical snippets. He wrote about all aspects of medicine: diagnosis, therapy, regimen, and the philosophy of medicine. He codified the Hippocratic doctrine of the humours, but also consolidated an experimental dimension to medicine. Whereas the Hippocratics were content with careful observation, Galen went much further, offering anatomical and physiological accounts of what happened in health and disease. He was big on ego-strength and seemed to assume that his was the last word on virtually everything. He cannot be blamed that most doctors for more than a thousand years agreed with him.

Humoralism served Galen very well at the bedside, explaining disease, but he also developed a complicated physiology to explain normal bodily function, which relied on spirits (pneuma) rather than humours. Within his model, food was taken into the stomach, whence it was turned into chyle. This chyle went to the liver via the portal vein, where it was converted into blood suffused with natural pneuma. Some of this blood then was conveyed to the heart. Part of the blood from the heart went to the lungs to nourish this essential organ. Other portions of the heart's blood passed through invisible pores from the right to the left ventricle, where it mixed with vital pneuma, acquired from the lungs and ultimately through breathing air. This vital blood then went via the aorta and carotid artery to the brain, where it had its last refinement, with animal pneuma, and then via the nerves to initiate motion and sensation.

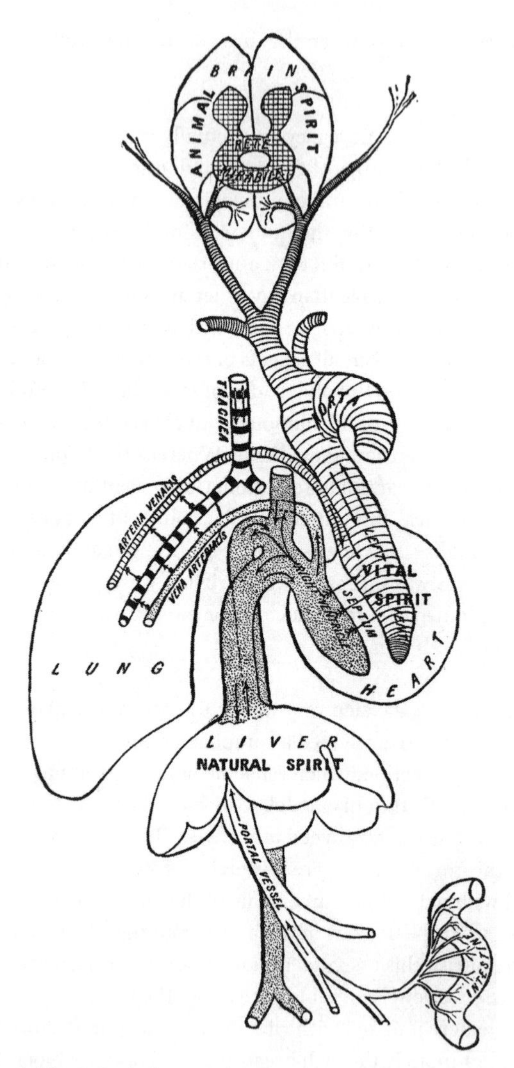

3. Galen's 'physiological system'. Galen accounted for many basic physiological phenomena by implicating the liver, heart, and brain in the elaboration and distribution of three kinds of 'spirit', the natural, vital, and animal

This model of human physiology became gospel for more than a millennium. So, too, did Galen's comments on anatomy, often (through no fault of his own) performed on pigs, apes, and other animals. The prohibition on human dissection was out of Galen's control, and his only mistake was not to tell his readers where he got his anatomical knowledge from. This omission encouraged later worshippers of Galen to assume that the human body must have changed since the master dissected, but eventually left him a sitting target for progressives who believed their own eyes.

More than 500 years separated Hippocrates and Galen, and there were of course many doctors and systems of treatment afoot between them. One group of doctors in Rome emphasized massage, warm or cool baths, and other therapies to relax or constrict the body's pores, their preternatural state of tension posited as the cause of disease. Other doctors adopted their own approach to diagnosis and treatment. Some of these alternative systems survived Galen's dominance, but Galen bestrode the millennium after his death far more comprehensively than Hippocrates had done in the centuries after his followers stopped writing. These medical dimensions are worth studying for their own sake, but Greek medicine as a whole left three basic principles that formed medicine until the modern period.

The first principle, as we have already seen, was humoralism. The second was the botanical basis of most drugs. Doctors looked to the botanical kingdom for medicines to combat disease. One doctor in particular organized the ancient pharmacopoeia into a form that others found useful for centuries. Dioscorides (fl. c. 40–80) wrote a treatise on *Materia Medica* which incorporated the medical-botanical writings of earlier authors but also included much that he himself had discovered about plants and their medicinal qualities. Although he described a few animal products, plants dominated, as they did for most other doctors in antiquity and beyond. Plants could yield substances that would bring on a sweat, induce vomiting or a purge, produce sleep, or control pain. Many botanical preparations, such as opium and hellebore, had great staying power, but unlike the core theoretical content of ancient medicine, plants have definite geographical distributions, and the search for them meant that later doctors had to do their own hunting, in their local forests and hedgerows. If you have a particular plant in your area, you can supply it to others who don't, and importing and exporting drugs became an active business in later centuries. Galen incorporated much of Dioscorides' work in his own voluminous writings, and the latter's *Materia Medica* was still prized in the Renaissance.

The third legacy – a secular approach to disease – was more elusive but just as important for all that. Both religion and magic continued to influence thinking about health and disease by doctors and laymen. They still do. But the ancient healers whose writings survived and were prized believed that disease could be understood in natural terms. This is not to say that ancient doctors were not religious: Galen had a notion of monotheism that later commentators turned into a kind of recognition of the religious movement that was gaining ground during his lifetime – Christianity. But when Hippocrates or Galen was confronted with a sick patient, they drew on their own knowledge and skills in an attempt to bring about an act of healing at the bedside. For all this, disease still frequently was and is experienced within a religious or moral framework, seen as a result of sin, punishment, or, like Job, trial – why me?

These glosses do not negate the fact that the framework of ancient medicine was a naturalistic one. Physician and physics derive from the same Greek root, meaning 'nature', and attempting to understand the way the body functions in health and disease has ever been a spur for the curious doctor and worried patient.

Chapter 2
Medicine in the library

The miracle of survival

When one stops to think about it, it is a miracle that anything written survives from antiquity. How is it that we can enjoy Homer's epic poems, Plato's and Aristotle's works, or the 20 volumes (in their incomplete modern edition) of Galen's writings? Manuscripts were laboriously copied by hand, on parchment or other mediums, were scarce and expensive commodities, and were then subjected to the ravages of time, the destruction of war, natural decay, or simple carelessness. The items that survive today are usually later copies, made centuries after the original text, prepared because someone wanted a version for himself. In general, the more prized a text was, the greater the chance of survival, simply because there were more versions of it made. But far more words written in antiquity have perished than have come down to us. The largest library and museum in the ancient world was in Alexandria, Egypt. It housed tens of thousands of scrolls and parchments, but suffered serial destruction and continuous decay from the 2nd century and was nothing but ruins by the 7th.

Thus, we are indebted to the anonymous scribes in great households, religious establishments, and royal courts for much of what we know of the thoughts of people who lived two millennia and more ago. The writings of Hippocrates, Galen, and other doctors of antiquity provided the formal foundations of medical practice into the 18th century. Consequently, the period of appreciation, preservation, and commentaries upon their works that characterizes the millennium between the fall of Rome in 455 and the movement we call the Renaissance deserves its own place in the history of medicine. It has been called the period of 'library medicine'. In this chapter, I shall make little distinction between the Latin West and the polyglot East, which includes Byzantium, the Islamic Empire, and Jewish and Christian contributions to medical life in the areas in which Islam came to dominate. Doctors in these widely separated geographical and cultural milieus all shared one characteristic: a veneration of the medical wisdom of the Greeks, and a desire to base their own medical theories and practices on these ancient precepts. Of course, they added much along the way.

Along with this essential contribution of preserving and adding to the Greek medical heritage, this epoch, from the 5th century to the invention of the printing press, also fundamentally changed the nature of medical structures. It bequeathed to us three important things: the hospital, the hierarchical division of medical practitioners, and the university, where the elites of medicine were educated.

Preservation, transmission, adaptation

In late antiquity Europe, medical care was mostly in the hands of individuals without access to any of the writings of the classical period. Local traditions, including informal care, magico-religious remedies, and superstitions dominated, but the prevailing world view of the Christian era encouraged individuals to wait for the end of the world, and in any case, to see disease as a part of a wider providence, and trivial compared to the potential joys of the world to come. The few literate doctors would have had access to some 4th- and 5th-century writings within the classical tradition.

Caelius Aurelianus (fl. 4th or early 5th century) produced a compilation on acute and chronic diseases, based largely on the works of an earlier physician, Soranus. Caelius's work was rational, full of medical insights, and survived throughout the medieval period as a summary of diseases and their treatments. For example, he described migraine, sciatica, and a number of common diseases. His treatments were mostly gentle, suggesting massage, bed rest, heat, and passive exercise for dealing with sciatica.

A few other medical works were also around in the Latin West: some minor works of Galen, including spurious treatises attributed to him, the Hippocratic *Aphorisms*, as well as bits of other ancient authors. The centre of gravity had shifted east, however, to the Byzantine Empire, the capital of which was Constantinople, now Istanbul. A lot of ancient manuscripts had already found their way east, and physicians in the Christian East preserved, translated, and commented on them. The rise of Islam saw Byzantium decline in influence and territory, but those same lands, now within Islamic dominion, were also significant for the transmission of the ancient corpus of medicine.

Islam was a wonderfully polyglot culture, and a number of Greek manuscripts survived only in the languages of the area of Islamic conquest, especially Arabic, Persian, and Syriac. A major translation movement was underway by the late 8th century, and this continued for three centuries. The medieval Islamic medical tradition is often seen primarily as a conduit for the preservation and transmission of ancient Greek texts, which were translated into the Middle Eastern languages, then in turn rendered back into Latin, and finally into modern European languages.

Medieval Islamic medicine was more than an interlude, however. There was also a vigorous learned medical culture which not only reformulated Greek medical ideas to its own context but also added new observations, medicaments, and procedures. Three of the great names of Islamic medicine, Rhazes (c. 865–925/32), Avicenna (980–1037), and Averroes (1126–98), span almost four centuries, and between them produced a corpus of work that assimilated Greek ideas and passed them, properly transformed, back to the West. All of them were men of wide interests. Rhazes, active in what is modern-day Iran, wrote on alchemy, music, and philosophy, but his actual medical practice was extensive, and his diagnostic acumen was much admired during his lifetime. He distinguished smallpox from measles for the first time (measles he judged the graver illness), and offered shrewd medical advice for travellers.

Like Rhazes, Avicenna (Ibn Sina) was a man with many interests outside of medicine. Aristotle was the dominant philosophical influence on him, and infused his medical writings. A precocious youth, Avicenna produced more than 250 titles in the course of an adventurous life. His *Canon of Medicine* (*Al-Qanum fi l-tibb*) has been described as the most studied medical treatise of all time, and its five Books cover the whole of medical theory, treatment, and hygiene, as well as associated surgical and pharmacological dimensions of medical practice. Like Galen, Avicenna was a clever man who did not hesitate to tell his readers about his talents, but the *Canon* brilliantly assimilates and packages Greek medical wisdom and Islamic medical experience, in a logical and well-ordered form. It was ideal as a complete medical textbook, for which it was long used in Europe, in Latin translation, and continues to be assigned to students of *unani tibb* (traditional Islamic) medicine.

Averroes (Ibn Rushd), like Avicenna well versed in Aristotelian philosophy, worked in Islamic Spain and in Morocco. His major medical work (he also published on philosophy, astronomy, and jurisprudence) was an encyclopaedic one, in the style of Avicenna's *Canon*. Variously rendered in English as 'The Book of Universals', or 'Generalities of Medicine', Averroes' textbook in seven sections covered the whole gamut of medicine, from anatomy to therapy. Its Latin translations presented a Galenic-Aristotelian synthesis to generations of doctors in late medieval Europe.

Just as the Islamic doctors had instituted a programme of translation of ancient texts into Middle Eastern languages, so the process of translating these translations back into Latin was initiated by Constantine the African (d. before 1098), and continued by many other scholars. These newly available Latin texts formed the basis of the curriculum of the earliest European medical schools, beginning with the famous one at Salerno, southern Italy, established about 1080, and adopted by medieval university medical faculties during the following centuries.

Hospitals, universities, doctors

Depending on what counts as a 'hospital', this central institution of modernity can be traced to various beginnings. The Romans used special buildings called *Valetudinaria* (from the same root as our word for someone who is worried well, a valetudinarian) to house and care for wounded and sick soldiers. There is one known to date from about CE 9. Slightly earlier, slaves were also being housed together when they were sick, a reflection of their value. These structures were pragmatically designed to contain a number of beds and related facilities, but they were also generally related to the necessity of a particular campaign or outbreak of illness and were not conceived of as permanent institutions in the modern sense.

Our word 'hospital' comes from the same root word as do hospitality, hostel, and hotel. In Christendom, early 'hospitals' were religious establishments, maintained by religious orders and available as places of refuge or hospitality for pilgrims, but also for the needy. Their function was not explicitly medical, although (like monasteries or nunneries) the 'hospital' might also contain an 'infirmary' (place for the sick or infirm), where those with specific medical needs could be looked after. More common and larger in the Near East (Jerusalem contained one with 200 beds by 550) than in the Latin West, they gradually began to dot the landscape of present-day Europe. Many of the famous European hospitals of the present date back to medieval times and their names testify to their religious origins: Hôtel Dieu in Paris, St Bartholomew's Hospital in London, Sta Maria Nuova in Florence.

Within the Islamic lands, hospitals also attained considerable size and importance by the 11th century. They sometimes had special divisions, such as wards for patients suffering from eye diseases, or the insane, and attracted students wishing to learn how to practise medicine. They were probably more overtly 'medical' than their Christian counterparts, but they shared the same range of philanthropic or charitable funding, and, in times of epidemic, the same function of isolation and segregation. Community leaders made use of hospitals for two diseases in particular: plague and leprosy. Often called 'lazarettos' – from Lazarus, the poor man whose sores the dogs licked in Jesus' parable in Luke's Gospel – these isolation hospitals were adapted for plague after the Black Death, from their earlier use for people diagnosed as lepers. No disease better than leprosy captures the combination of brutality and love infusing medieval Christendom. The diagnosis itself, often for conditions that modern doctors would give another name, carried with it total social ostracism and legal death, with divorce by the leper's spouse permitted. It condemned its victim to a life of isolation and begging, generally confined to a lazaretto and needing to carry the familiar leper's rattle when going outside, so that passers-by were alerted to the oncoming source of physical (and moral) contagion. At the same time, some monks, nuns, and other religiously motivated individuals freely lived among these outcasts and devoted their lives to them.

The leprosy diagnosis was common from the 12th to the 14th centuries, in most parts of Europe, and leprosy's decline may have

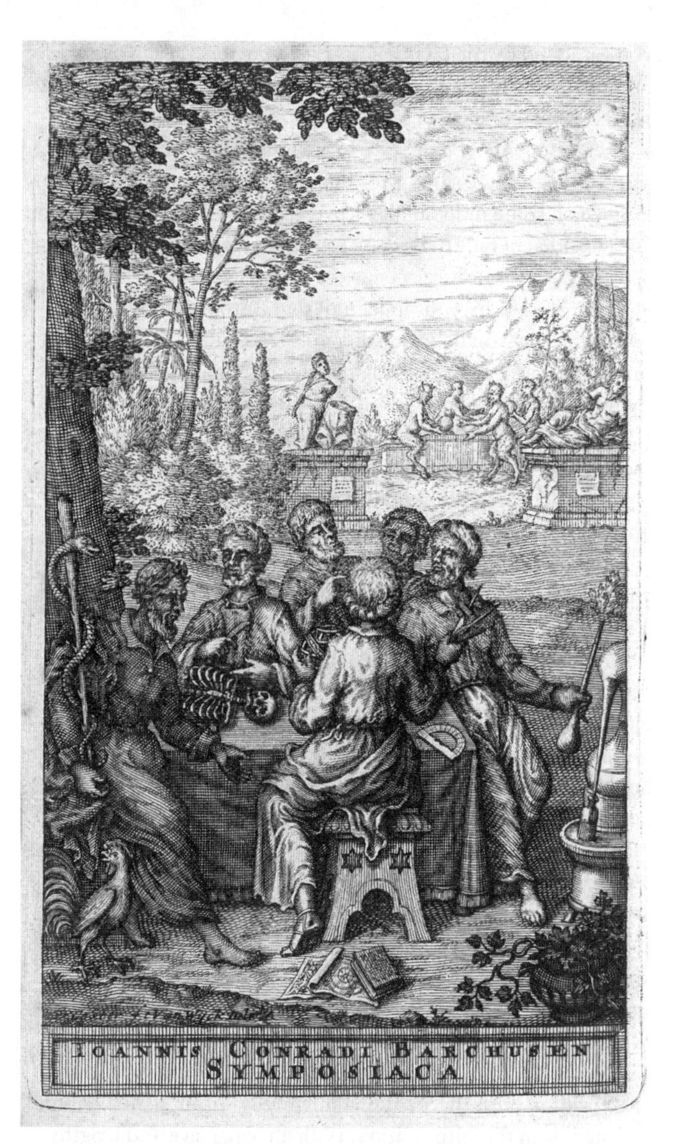

4. Classical medical figures. This early-modern image, in the classical style, depicts Asclepius on the left, holding a caduceus, and Galen examining a skeleton

been catalysed by the fact that people living together in closely confined quarters were particularly vulnerable to the Black Death and the repeated plague epidemics that followed. Certainly a number of leper hospitals were turned into plague hospitals, for many of the same reasons, save that plague was an acute disease, from which some individuals recovered, and leprosy was a chronic disease and generally a life-long sentence. Plague hospitals, especially in southern Europe, were converted to other medical uses after that disease disappeared from Europe in the 17th century; in the Middle East, where plague continued, they were kept as places for quarantining travellers and others on the move when plague was near.

Another medieval institution important for medicine was the university. The medical school at Salerno from the late 11th century was simply that: a school to train doctors. A university followed there a couple of centuries later. In the meantime, many others were founded throughout Europe, beginning with Bologna (founded c. 1180), and followed by those in Paris (1200), Oxford (1200), and Salamanca (c. 1218). By the late 15th century, there were 50 in Europe, dotting the north and south, east and west. A university has different faculties, and most of these either had from the beginning or developed medical faculties, to complement those of arts, philosophy (including what we would call science), theology, and law. Although many of the medical faculties were very small, and the number of graduates miniscule, the movement gave birth to learned medicine, and the university-educated physician. It represented the quintessence of 'library medicine', since the teaching was initially based on texts, of classical and Islamic authors, and disputation rather than practical training or experiment was the key.

One consequence of the newly graduated physician was the formalization of the occupational hierarchy within medicine that persisted until the 19th century. With an expensive and lengthy education that the universities offered came the gentlemanly status that physicians long prided themselves on. (Until a decade ago, Fellows of the Royal College of Physicians of London could not sue for the recovery of fees.) As gentlemen, manual work was beneath them. That was the job of the surgeon and apothecary, both occupational niches that already existed but were more formally fixed with the coming of the university. Surgeons and apothecaries were trained by apprenticeships, or by informally learning their craft by associating themselves with an older practitioner. It was the Hippocratic way, but it began to acquire a lower social (and, generally, economic) status when compared with physicians who could read Latin and dispute the niceties of Galen and Avicenna.

There were, to be sure, a few surgeons with university exposure, and among both surgeons and apothecaries, individuals with learning and wealth. The boundaries were not always fixed and, in the countryside, many physicians compounded their own drugs and performed surgery. In other words, they acted as general practitioners. In urban areas, however, the divisions were retained and regulated by colleges and companies of physicians, or by the university faculty. Surgeons in urban areas often established guilds, on a par with those regulating other manual occupations, such as butchering, baking, or candlestick making. The medical regulation was patchy, but the image of the three occupational hierarchies remained part of public perception until later developments in medical knowledge also changed what doctors could do.

The discovery of anatomy

Galen and a number of other ancient and Arabic authors had had a good deal to say on the internal structures and functions of the human body. Since then, the occasional autopsy, mostly performed when an important person died suddenly or in suspicious circumstances, had revealed more of what the body looks like when it is cut open. For all that, it was a bold step when the

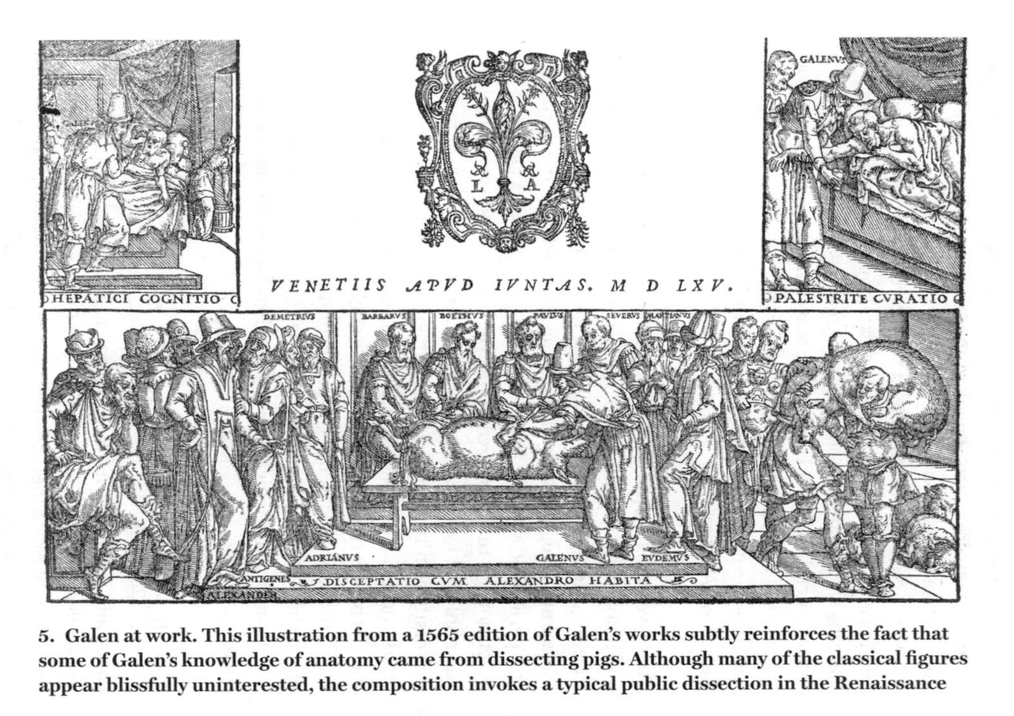

5. Galen at work. This illustration from a 1565 edition of Galen's works subtly reinforces the fact that some of Galen's knowledge of anatomy came from dissecting pigs. Although many of the classical figures appear blissfully uninterested, the composition invokes a typical public dissection in the Renaissance

medical faculties gradually began to offer public demonstrations of dissected bodies in the 14th century. Frequently, a menial prosector would open the corpse (often of an executed criminal) while the professor read relevant passages from Galen or another authority. These 'anatomies', as the whole process was called, were scheduled for the winter months, when the colder weather slowed down the body's putrefaction; the order of exposing the internal parts was also dictated by the speed of decay: abdomen first, followed by the contents of the thorax, then the brain, and finally, the limbs.

The first recorded public dissection was performed in Bologna in about 1315, by Mondino de' Liuzzi (c. 1270–1326), who also wrote the first modern book devoted to anatomy, in about 1316. It took almost a century for dissections to become relatively common, a combination of the difficulty of obtaining corpses, and the theoretical bias of most medical education. From the 15th century, however, the pace quickened, with more dissections and more works devoted to human anatomy. Renaissance artists wanted to appreciate what the human body looked like on both the outside and inside; Leonardo da Vinci's (1452–1519) anatomical drawings are some of the most famous of the period, although they had remained virtually unknown, and therefore without influence.

The greatest of the early anatomists was Andreas Vesalius (1514–64), Belgium born but professor of anatomy and surgery in Padua. His great work *De humani corporis fabrica* (1543: 'On the fabric of the human body') is the first medical book in which the illustrations are more important than the text.

What Vesalius, himself an ardent dissector rather than simply a reader of Galen, had noticed was that the human body was not always as Galen had described it. While others had done so before, Vesalius not only said so – diffidently at first, more forcefully as he gained confidence – but he demonstrated it

DE HVMANI CORPORIS FABRICA LIBER VII. 617

DVODECIMA SEPTIMI LIBRI FIGVRA.

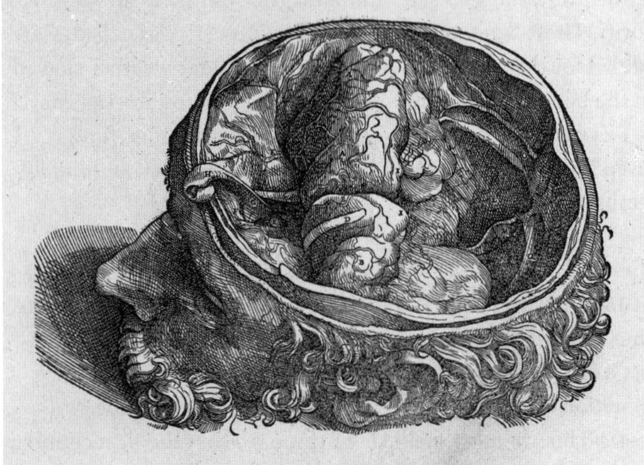

DVODECIMAE FIGVRAE, EIVSDEMQVE CHA-racterum Index.

6. In addition to the famous muscle-men, Vesalius's *Fabrica* of 1543 depicted other parts of the human body, always dramatically represented

through the magnificent plates that accompanied his large book. The muscular walls between the right and left side of the heart, for instance, were dense, with no way for blood to pass through, as Galen's physiology required. The human liver did not have the four or five lobes that Galen assigned it (through dissecting pigs and other animals); the sternum, uterus, and many other anatomical structures were accurately described by Vesalius for the first time.

We divide the history of anatomy into pre-Vesalian and post-Vesalian, with Vesalius as the fulcrum. This probably exaggerates the immediate impact of Vesalius' book, for he left Padua and anatomy shortly after its publication for a lucrative job at the Spanish court. By the mid-16th century, however, the anatomical revolution was well underway, and the desire to see for oneself, instead of taking the ancients on childlike trust, was widespread.

Anatomy was the queen of the medical sciences for some three centuries, and no branch of medical knowledge benefited more from that catalyst of social and intellectual change, the printing press. A German artisan, Johannes Gutenberg (c. 1400–68), introduced the movable type printing press into Europe in about 1439 (the Chinese already had them). The impact on all aspects of human life was enormous. Medical books were well represented in the early incunabula (books printed before 1501), although Bibles, works of theology, and editions and translations of ancient authors dominated. Books could then be mass-produced, and even ordinary doctors could own a few of them.

In addition to the texts, woodcuts and engravings allowed books to be illustrated, so not only could people read about the human body, they could see its parts displayed on the page. Vesalius' *De Fabrica* was not the first illustrated anatomy text, but it set standards for dramatic artistic representation as well as anatomical accuracy. Over the following centuries, anatomy books crystallize a deep paradox in early-modern medicine. Anatomy was an aspect of medical activity that attracted revulsion from many members of the public: dissecting was seen as morally debasing, disgusting, and cruel. It led eventually to an underground trade in the supply of bodies by illegal means, generally grave-robbing but sometimes murder. It certainly was smelly before preservation methods improved, although the sickly sweet aroma of formaldehyde made modern medical students easy to identify on the street, permeating as it does their clothes and skin.

Dissection was thus bad for medicine's public image. It was also the subject of elaborate, expensive, and beautifully produced and

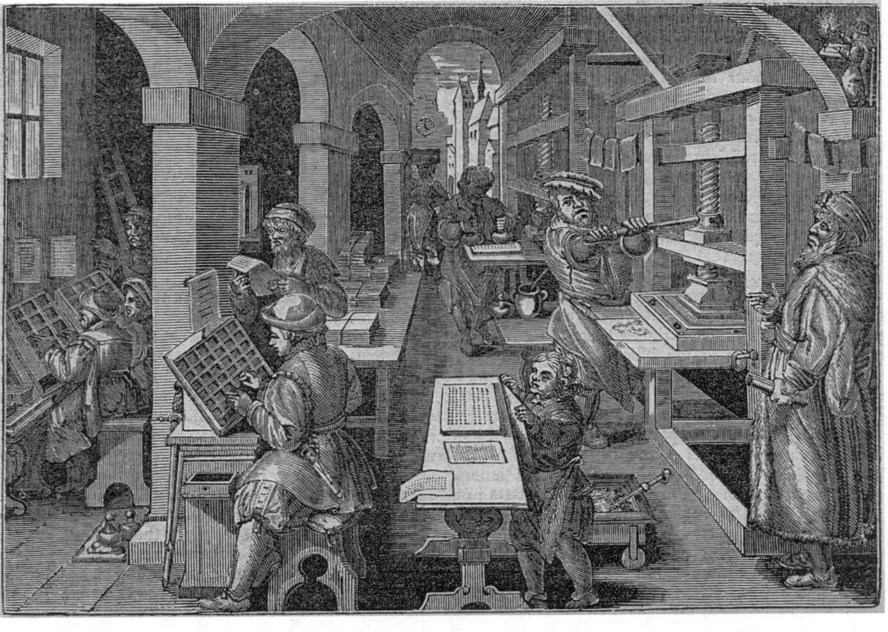

7. This Victorian engraving of a woodcut by Stradanus from about 1580 shows many stages of book production, including setting type, inking it, printing the sheets, and proof-reading

illustrated books, with the upper end of the market aimed at the connoisseur. For the medical student, there were small textbooks with crude illustrations and a price to match. No other discipline within medicine so combined art and science, or knowledge and presentation. Increasingly, even would-be physicians dissected, their curiosity getting the better of their gentlemanly pretensions. Many of the great names in early-modern anatomy – Gabriele Fallopio (1532–62), Fabricius ab Acquapendente (1533–1619), Frederik Ruysch (1638–1731), William Cheselden (1688–1752), William Hunter (1718–83) – had affiliations with surgery or obstetrics, but curious physicians, such as William Harvey (1578–1657), also used their hands in their research. Harvey's great treatise announcing his discovery of the circulation of the blood (1628) is actually entitled an 'anatomical exercise' on *de Motu Cordis* (On the motion of the heart).

Given the nature of medical (or even surgical) practice in the period, doctors learned more anatomy than they could actually use. But the parts of the body were palpable and it was easier to agree on an anatomical structure than on some theoretical nicety. And anatomy was a discipline in which progress was discernible. New parts were regularly being described, such as the lacteal vessels, the valves of the veins, or the 'circle of Willis' – the arterial anastomosis at the base of the brain, named after Thomas Willis (1621–75). By the early 17th century, few anatomists would have deferred to Galen, and in the 'battle of the books', that widespread debate covering all fields of natural knowledge about whether the ancients or the moderns know the most about the world we inhabit, anatomy was one field in which the moderns won hands-down.

The chemical, the physical, and the clinical

The liberation effected by the injunction to look for oneself touched many aspects of medicine as well as natural philosophy. The Renaissance coincided with the period that later historians have named the Scientific Revolution, which influenced medicine as well as astronomy, cosmology, physics, and other sciences. The two natural sciences that most closely impinged on medicine were chemistry and physics.

The chemical movement within medicine had its roots in an eccentric Swiss genius, Paracelsus (c. 1493–1541). Paracelsus was how he was known to his followers: his full name, Theophrastus Philippus Aureolus Bombastus von Hohenheim, was something of a mouthful. The story that he meant his adopted name to mean 'greater than Celsus', the Roman author who wrote an influential compendium on medicine, is probably mythical, but it embodies one of two particularly striking and influential characteristics of his chequered career. He was passionate about the fact that medicine (and science) needed to be founded again on first principles, by the moderns. He had little use for the wisdom of Hippocrates or Galen, publicly burning one of the latter's books in a defiant display during a (brief) stint as a professor in Basel. Although he probably never converted to the new Protestantism, Paracelsus was obviously influenced by the intellectual and emotional ferment that Martin Luther's movement formally inaugurated early in his life. Paracelsus repeatedly said that learning was to be found in nature, not books, although this did not stop him from penning dozens of books himself, many of which were printed in his lifetime. Perhaps he really meant that learning was to be found in *his* books, not those of his predecessors.

His second lasting contribution was his emphasis on chemistry, as a way of understanding the way the human body works, and as a source of drugs to treat disease. He used metals such as mercury and arsenic as much as the traditional botanicals in his treatments, and his followers, the iatrochemists (literally, chemical doctors), continued in his wake. His notion of disease, as something external to the body, is sometimes rather inappropriately described as a forerunner of germ theory, but it was in fact rooted in his mystical, alchemical notions of the way nature operates. There is more to the thinking of this strange man, who provoked controversy in his lifetime and afterwards. His followers, of which there were many for well over a century, attempted to rewrite the theory and practice of medicine, in a chemical language.

Another group, the iatrophysicists, slightly later and drawing on the triumphs of astronomy and physics, saw the body as a wonderful mechanical contrivance. Whereas the iatrochemists considered digestion as a chemical process, the iatrophysicists saw it as a mechanical grinding down. These later advocates analysed muscular movement, calculating the forces generated by contraction, and sought to represent human physiology mathematically whenever possible. Their heroes were Galileo, and later Newton, men who had replaced Aristotle's view of the universe with a much more powerful model, in which matter and force were the operative things to be measured. Throughout the 18th century, Newton's notion of gravity as a force that extended throughout the universe and explained so much was a spur to doctors seeking similar principles in medicine.

The new relationship to enquiry introduced a period of great ferment within medicine (and science). Theories abounded and optimism prevailed. The approach to understanding health and disease altered dramatically, but changes in what doctors actually did in treating patients were less striking. To be sure, the chemicals introduced by Paracelsus and his followers were mostly new, and the prevalence of syphilis meant that mercury had a prominent medical presence. Syphilis had taken Europe by storm in the 1490s. Appearing first in Naples, where some of the Spanish mercenaries had been to the New World with Columbus, the assumption that it was a new disease imported with Columbus was a natural conclusion. Historians are still debating this scenario, but the fact remains that syphilis in the late 14th and early 15th centuries behaved like a new disease, in its virulence and rapidity of spread. Because of the rash caused by syphilis, mercury, a standard treatment for skin diseases, was used, and it seemed effective in suppressing symptoms, even if it was toxic for the sufferer, producing intense salivation, loss of teeth, and other side effects. The metallic odour to the patient's breath was difficult to conceal, and although popes, artists, and doctors suffered from it, its sexual transmission was suspected early on (the genital lesions were usually the first sign), and the introduction of the bark of the guaiacum tree, from South America, soon became the favoured therapy for those who could afford it. It reinforced the notion that syphilis had come from the

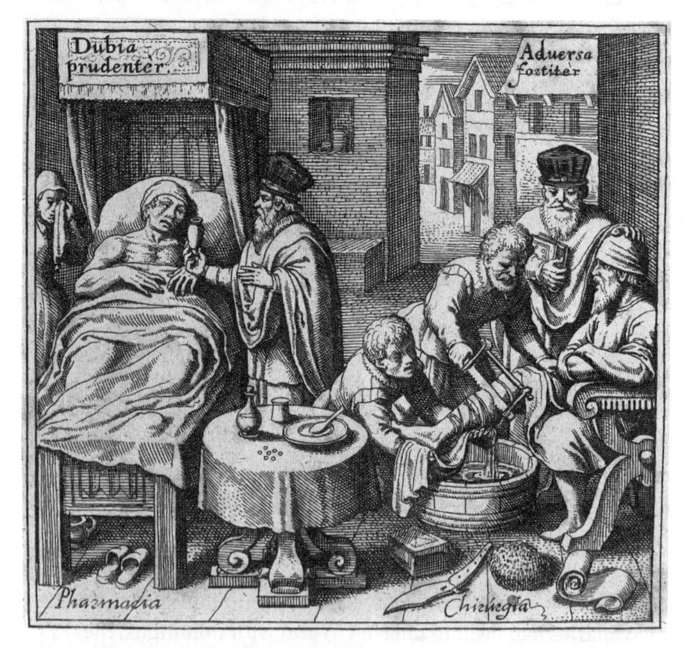

8. The differing social status and medical functions of the physician and surgeon are shown in this engraving from 1646. In these two scenes, the formally dressed physician on the left hands a medicine to a sick man in bed; on the right, he supervises the more roughly attired surgeon who is amputating a man's leg

New World, the assumption being that God placed remedies near to the origins of diseases, to encourage us to look for them.

Despite these new diseases and new remedies, Hippocrates would not have been surprised at most medical ministration to sufferers. Bloodletting, emetics (to invoke vomiting), cathartics (to induce purging), and the gamut of remedies associated with humoralism continued as the mainstay of doctors. Indeed, as Galen's star waned, that of Hippocrates still shone brightly. Among clinicians of the 17th century, Thomas Sydenham (1624–89) still commands respect. Called the 'English Hippocrates', he sought to return medicine to the empirical art that he identified with the Father of medicine. Medicine, he wrote, should concern itself with careful clinical descriptions of disease (he left graphic accounts of gout, hysteria, and smallpox, among other illnesses). With the security of correctly diagnosing a disease, remedies could be empirically sought. He was instrumental in advocating another New World remedy, quinine (variously called Peruvian bark, or Jesuit's bark, reflecting its origin), in the treatment of intermittent fevers.

Sydenham's experience with Peruvian bark fundamentally changed his whole concept of disease. Although he was still comfortable with Hippocratic humours, quinine seemed completely to stamp out intermittent fevers, root and branch. It seemed to be a *specific*, dramatically effective against this one disorder in all patients. It encouraged him to believe that diseases could be classified, like botanists classify plants, and that the variation of a disease and its symptoms in individuals was adventitious, like the differences in individual violets or other flowers. As he famously wrote:

> Nature, in the production of disease, is uniform and consistent, so much so, that for the same disease in different persons the symptoms are for the most part the same; and the selfsame phenomena that you would observe in the sickness of a Socrates you would observe in the sickness of a simpleton.

Sydenham's reflection can be seen as a kind of turning point in clinical thinking. It encouraged doctors in the generations that followed to classify diseases; more significantly, it began the modern process of teasing out the difference between the disease and the person suffering from the disease, and of identifying those universal features of each kind of disease that could make a specific therapy rational. The irony is, Sydenham never saw himself as anything but a good Hippocratic, but his thinking had posed the modern medical dilemma: how to retain a belief in the unique individuality of each patient, and still apply the more general findings of a scientifically grounded diagnosis and therapy.

Enlightened medicine?

Sydenham enjoyed a good reputation in the century that followed his death. His works were originally published in Latin, still the lingua franca, but also appeared in many translated editions, in English, French, German, Spanish, and other European languages. The most famous medical teacher of the 18th century, Hermann Boerhaave (1668–1738), reputedly never mentioned Sydenham in his lectures without lifting his hat in salute. Boerhaave was the leading light at the University of Leiden for more than 40 years, and his pupils came from all over Europe, and influenced educational initiatives in Edinburgh, Vienna, Göttingen, Geneva, and elsewhere.

Boerhaave was intellectually an eclectic, drawing his medical ideas from chemistry, physics, botany, and other disciplines, but also possessing a wonderful common sense and diagnostic acumen. Both his lectures and his bedside teaching were famous, and he had an extensive private practice, including, as was still common, a large postal consultation, both with puzzled doctors and worried patients. Equally important, Boerhaave wrote a string of textbooks in chemistry, materia medica (i.e. medical therapeutics), and medicine, as well as numerous publications in anatomy, botany,

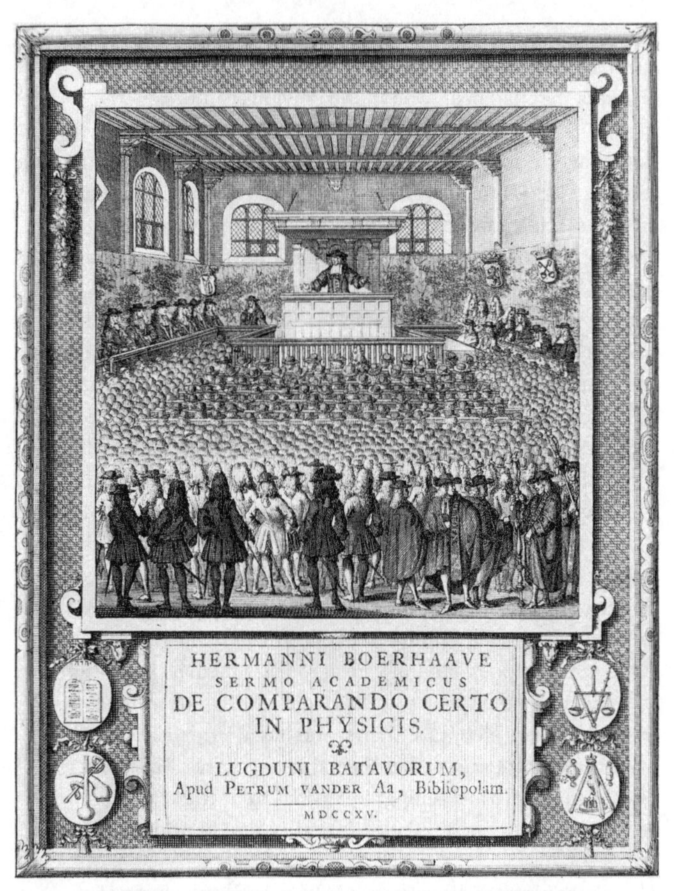

9. Hermann Boerhaave was the most famous medical teacher of his day, and although he trained many young doctors, he probably did not often lecture to quite such large audiences

and venereal disease. He influenced two or three generations of doctors, even if his forte was synthesis rather than fundamental discovery. Despite his fascination with the natural world (especially his beloved botanical garden), he remains a part of the learned tradition of library medicine: Hippocrates was still a vital figure for him, and he continued to look back for facts and approaches to medicine, even while retaining the confidence in progress that had been won in the previous century.

Boerhaave's pupils included the most famous naturalist of the 18th century, Carl Linnaeus (1707–78). Linnaeus turned classification into an avant-garde science, introducing the system of binomial nomenclature, whereby organisms are known by their genus and species. Linnaeus devoted his life to ordering the objects of the natural world, especially plants. He saw himself as a second Adam, the first having been charged with the task of naming the animals and plants in the Garden of Eden. Uppsala, where Linnaeus was professor of medicine, was no Eden, but he orchestrated a series of expeditions by his students to many exotic parts of the world from which they dutifully brought back (if they survived) natural specimens of all kinds for him to classify. Linnaeus also produced a classification of diseases, but his nosology was less influential than several other Enlightenment ones, including those of François Boissier de la Croix de Sauvages (1706–67) of Montpellier, William Cullen (1710–90) of Edinburgh, and Erasmus Darwin (1731–1802), a poet, botanist, inventor, and medical practitioner in Lichfield and other places in the English Midlands. All these nosologies were elaborate affairs, and based primarily on what we would call symptoms, rather than signs or causes. Fever was a disease in itself. Most tellingly, pain was minutely classified, according to its characteristics, intensity, and location.

These mappings of disease revealed a prominent aspect of Enlightenment medicine, in that it was patient-orientated, thus continuing the Hippocratic tradition. Doctors relied on patients' accounts of their own feelings and symptoms to make their diagnoses, and within this scenario, patients are generally described by historians as dominating the encounter. It is possible to exaggerate this, just as it is possible to describe the medicine of the 19th century and beyond as universally doctor-dominated. Nevertheless, before the diagnostic methods of modern times, patients would not have taken away from their encounter the bad news that their blood pressure or blood sugar was too high (or too low), or that there was a suspicious shadow on a chest X-ray. In the *ancien régime*, patients and their doctors spoke the same language and had similar conceptions of disease and its causes. They might go away with a grave or a favourable prognosis, but it would have been directly related to the symptoms that led them to seek medical advice in the first place.

Two further aspects of Enlightenment medical practice ought to be mentioned. First, it was a time of impressive medical entrepreneurialism. Health mattered, and people were prepared to pay for it. This meant that ambitious (or devious) healers of all stripes could seek to carve out their niche in the medical market place. Telling the difference between the 'quacks' and the 'regulars' was not always easy, since many so-called quacks also generally operated within the cultural cosmology of medicine, and 'regulars' might advertise their therapies, use secret remedies, and cultivate notoriety as a means of attracting attention, and thereby patients. The complementary medicine of the present, based as it usually is on an alternative set of causal explanations of health and disease, had little resonance in earlier centuries. Individual quacks might have had their own idiosyncratic notions of what caused disease, or how it might best be treated, but as often as not they would also assimilate important historical figures within medicine – Hippocrates and Galen both feature in the advertisements of irregular healers of the period. Paracelsus is a notable exception, in rejecting not only the theories but also the whole tradition of medicine. His was a genuinely ahistorical mentality; most 'quacks' relied instead on the familiar and traditional, slyly turning it to their own advantage, in what they promised or in how they plied their wares and services.

The second striking characteristic of Enlightenment medicine was its busy optimism. It was an age of projects and institutions. Hospitals were established with great regularity, attempts were made throughout Europe to reform military medical services, and medically orientated philanthropy was common. The idea of progress, including medical progress, was taken for granted, and doctors and their patients both believed that the medicine of the future could do even more than the medicine of the past or present. At the same time, learned physicians and surgeons still looked to Hippocrates or Sydenham, not simply for inspiration but for information and example. For Boerhaave or Cullen, the history of medicine was not of mere antiquarian interest, but a source of living wisdom. During the 19th century, the old doctors were consigned to history, as a new generation of doctors began increasingly to look to the future.

Chapter 3
Medicine in the hospital

Vive la France

The phrase 'hospital medicine' has acquired a specific meaning for medical historians. Hospitals emerged in the early medieval period, and 'medicine', in the sense of medical practice, has an even longer history. Nevertheless, 'hospital medicine' is a convenient shorthand for the values that flourished within the medical community in France, and especially Paris, between the revolutions of 1789 and 1848. This period constitutes an epoch, during which Paris became the Mecca of the medical world. It was centred squarely within the Parisian hospitals and the tools and attitudes that dominated medical education and practice there resonated throughout the Western world.

This French period has sometimes been described as a 'medical revolution', appropriate since it grew out of a political revolution. Historians who have minutely unpacked the educational structures, medical procedures, and doctor–patient relationships have uncovered sufficient precedent to argue for evolution rather than revolution within medicine, but the fact remains that doctors in the 1840s had acquired a new confidence, when compared to their predecessors a couple of generations before, and much of this can be ascribed to the influence of Paris.

Like many revolutions, the Parisian medical one began small, and could have hardly been predicted during the turbulent days of the Terror. As the political and military forces of the Revolution gained power, the institutions of medicine – physicians, surgeons, hospitals, the old academies and faculties – were swept away, along with the other detritus of the *Ancien Régime*. For a couple of heady years in the early 1790s, it seemed best for everyone to be his or her own doctor, and revolutionary leaders promised that universal health would inevitably follow the abolition of privilege and corruption associated with the old hierarchies and inequalities.

The optimism did not last long. Disease did not disappear, and the Revolutionary government soon discovered that its soldiers and sailors demanded medical care when they were sick or wounded. The army needed its doctors, and, more particularly, doctors trained in both medicine and surgery. The old dichotomy was inefficient in the midst of campaigns and battles, and in 1794, three medical schools were reopened, primarily to produce men to serve the military needs of the new republic.

Fortunately, the key man on the commission appointed by the Revolutionary Assembly to consider the medical requirements of the new era was a doctor and chemist sympathetic to the aims of the Revolution. Antoine Fourcroy (1755–1809) had made his name as a chemist, and served as professor of chemistry in the new Parisian school he helped create. Politically astute and genuinely well-meaning, he masterminded the blueprint for the schools in Paris, Strasbourg, and Montpellier. The report he largely produced recognized the military needs of the contemporary political situation and stressed three aspects of the new medical education. First, it ought to be intensely practical from the first day of the student's training. In his ringing words, the student ought to 'read little, see much, do much'. No theory and much practice were the orders of the day. Second, the new medical education was to be

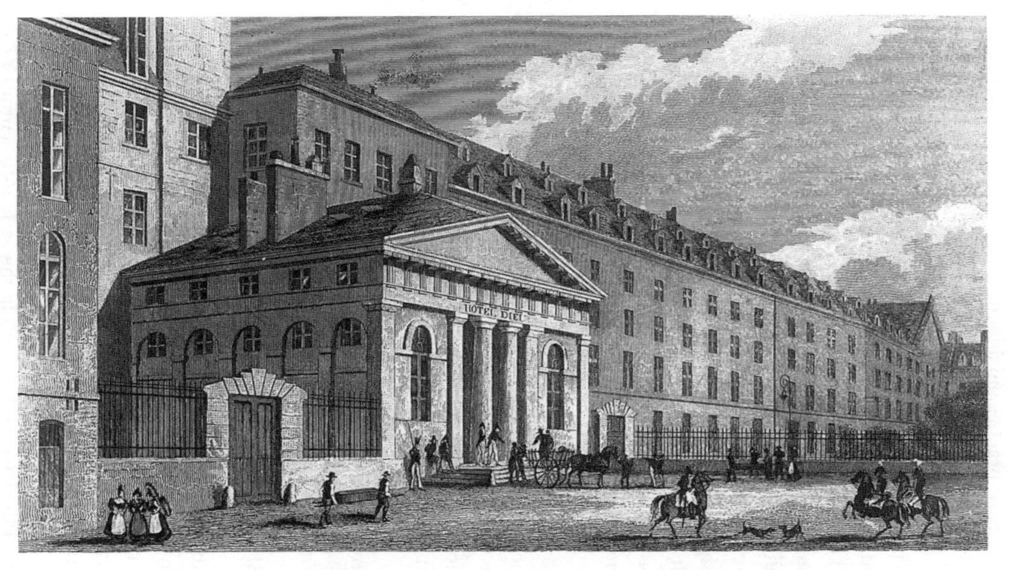

10. The massive edifice of the Hôtel Dieu Hospital, Paris, in the early 19th century, scene of so much medical innovation. The two figures on the left seem to be bearing a coffin, and the cart in front of the entrance may well be preparing to take away bodies for burial

based squarely within the hospital, where the opportunities for experience were much greater and more intense than in the lecture theatre or practice outside the hospital. Finally, the new medical graduate should be trained in both medicine and surgery. In effect, this meant the importation of surgical thinking into medicine proper. Whereas physicians had traditionally been concerned with the whole body, with humours, spirits, or other generalist conceptions of disease, surgeons had always been confronted with the local: with abscesses, broken bones, specific abnormalities requiring definitive intervention at a particular site. With the rise of the French medical schools, the *lesion* acquired medical significance. A lesion is a pathological change, induced by disease. It could thus be seen, either with or without a microscope. Physicians learned to think surgically, and the solid parts of the body came into their own within medicine.

French hospital medicine came to be based on three pillars, none entirely new, but which together constituted a new way of looking at disease. The three pillars were physical diagnosis, pathologico-clinical correlation, and the use of large numbers of cases to elucidate diagnostic categories and to evaluate therapy.

With many modifications, these have remained fundamental to medicine, as has the centrality of the hospital.

Physical diagnosis: the new intimacy

An encounter with a doctor has its own etiquette and intimacy. He or she can ask the patient to undress, can touch and feel in ways generally reserved for spouses or partners, and can cause discomfort. For the past two centuries or so, most patients have accepted this relationship with doctors, on the assumption that this dependency is for their own good. The relationship became routinized in the Parisian hospitals in the early 19th century, as a consequence of the physical examination that doctors developed in the newly opened hospital medical schools.

This is not to suggest that doctors, always male until the late 19th century, had never examined naked patients before. The vaginal speculum, for instance, was developed in Roman times, and operations for bladder stones or anal fistulae, the treatment of genital lesions, or deliveries of babies by male practitioners had occurred with some regularity in earlier centuries. Nevertheless, most medical encounters did not involve much physical contact with the doctor, other than his feeling the pulse and looking at the tongue. Bodily excretions such as the urine and faeces might also figure in medical diagnoses, but the doctor sometimes examined these without ever seeing his patient.

The doctor–patient encounter shifted in the Parisian hospitals of the early 19th century. Hospital patients were mostly the poor and uneducated, and therefore powerless to have much say in the way they were treated. Further, the new medical ideology encouraged doctors to look for objective signs of disease, rather than simply rely on the patient's account of his or her symptoms. A symptom, such as pain or tiredness, is private to the individual; signs, such as muscle wasting or an abscess, are more public matters, and the leaders of French hospital medicine wanted to base their practice on the objectivity of signs and lesions.

Physical diagnosis was central to this endeavour. The four cardinal dimensions of physical diagnoses, still taught to medical students, are inspection, palpation, percussion, and auscultation. In various forms, all had been used occasionally by doctors since the Hippocratics. The French hospital doctors put them together, made them routine and systematic, and forever changed doctor–patient relationships.

Inspection is the most basic: look at the patient. 'Stick out your tongue' has been a familiar medical command for ages. Furred tongues were deemed to be the key to fevers and other acute disorders. Yellow eyeballs pointed to jaundice, and flushed faces also indicated fevers or the end stages of a 'hectic' (a late stage of consumption, or tuberculosis), or the plethora of gout. A green tint to a pale face made the doctor think of chlorosis, a disease of young girls which mysteriously disappeared in the early 20th century, about the same time as hysteria, and possibly for the same reasons. For the most part, however, inspection was confined to the 'public' parts of our bodies: the face, hands, and other parts exposed without breech of convention. When a doctor looked elsewhere, there had to be a good reason, and surgeons were more likely to have a reason than physicians.

The French made inspection systematic, part of a general assessment of a patient's health. They did the same thing for palpation, an even more intimate manoeuvre, since it involves touching. A tender spot, lump, or enlarged organ can sometimes be observed, but it can more often be felt. The Hippocratics knew that intermittent fevers often produced an enlarged spleen, occasionally so prominent that it could be seen, but more often it could be detected by palpation. Within the gentlemanly culture of physicians in the early-modern period, however, probing the patient's body with one's hands smacked of manual labour. Palpation was thus another aspect of diagnosis imported back into medicine by the French injunction to integrate medicine and surgery. By locating disease processes within the organs, and emphasizing the importance of the lesion, French medical students were taught to use their hands as part of their diagnostic tools.

Percussion (tapping the chest or abdomen) was the third part of routine physical examination. Despite isolated comments in earlier case histories, the Viennese physician Leopold Auenbrugger (1722–1809) was within his rights when he called his 1761 treatise on the technique *Inventum novum* (New Discovery). The son of an innkeeper, the young Auenbrugger reputedly learned the value of percussion when, sent by his father to the cellar to discover how much wine and beer were left in the casks, he discovered the technique while tapping on the sides. At the point of the fluid level, the sound changed. This meant he did not have to take off the covers and peer, with the aid of a candle, into the barrels. As a practising physician, he adopted the procedure, to help determine when the heart, liver, or any other organ was enlarged, or when accumulations of fluids in the chest or abdomen meant that normally resonant body cavities were changed through disease.

Auenbrugger's modest little volume is an excellent example of the fact that classics are made, not born. It was barely noticed after publication, and only a handful of references to it in the following four decades have been recovered by historians. Doctors of the 18th century were simply not attuned to worrying too much about the solid parts of the body to aid their diagnoses. All this changed with the coming of the French way of teaching and learning medicine.

Auenbrugger's Latin treatise was rediscovered by Jean-Nicolas Corvisart (1755–1821), Napoleon's private physician and professor of medicine in the Paris school. Corvisart was well attuned to the new organ-based orientation of early 19th-century French medicine, and particularly interested in diseases of the heart. He recognized the value of percussion in cases of heart enlargement, collections of fluid around the heart, and other cardiac diseases. He began teaching percussion to his students and translated Auenbrugger's treatise in 1808 into French, adding extensive notes that quadrupled its length. His notes made it very clear how important this new technique could be in assisting the doctor in diagnoses. Two years earlier, his treatise on heart diseases had been published, largely through notes taken by one of his pupils. The case histories in this innovative volume make sober reading: Corvisart pessimistically concluded that organic diseases of the heart could rarely be effectively treated with the therapies available to him. It could be diagnosed, however, and one gets a spectrum of the patients in the Parisian hospitals from these histories: working-class men and women with grave disease, forced to seek the sanctuary of the hospital as a last resort. Mortality rates in the Paris hospitals were very high, and hospitals then were sometimes seen as 'gateways to death'.

To Corvisart's popularization of percussion was added the fourth, and most innovative, diagnostic tool: mediate auscultation. Doctors had sometimes listened to sounds coming from within their patients' bodies. Wheezing can be heard by other people, and not simply the individual having difficulty breathing; some heart murmurs are so loud that they can also be audible to others; an over-active intestine makes prominent noises. Sounds like these provide clues to what is going on inside a person's body, and they had been noted by doctors for hundreds of years. Occasionally, doctors had noted that they had put their ears directly on the patient's chest or abdomen, the better to hear. This is *immediate* auscultation, listening directly with the ear. *Mediate* auscultation involved something between the patient's body and the doctor's ear. This was the stethoscope, the invention of R. T. H. Laennec (1781–1826), one of the most complex and gifted of the French clinicians.

Laennec's career well illustrates the importance of external considerations in who's in and who's out. As a Catholic and Royalist, his career languished during the secular atmosphere that permeated the Republic and Napoleonic epochs. A hospital appointment and, eventually, a chair came only after the fall of Napoleon and the restoration of the monarchy. He had already imbibed the ideals of the French school, and contributed much as a journalist, editor, and practising doctor. His original stethoscope was no more than a tightly rolled notebook, constructed because he wanted to listen to the chest sounds of a plump young woman, and decorum meant that he could not place his ear directly on her chest. He was delighted to discover that the sound was transmitted even more clearly than it would have been had he employed immediate auscultation. He quickly devised a simple stethoscope (his word), a hollow wooden tube, with two fittings at the end, a bell and a diaphragm, the better to reproduce sounds of different pitches (he was a skilled musician).

His encounter with his female patient occurred in 1816, at the Necker Hospital, in Paris. Laennec's three years between 1816 and 1819 constitute one of the most creative periods for any individual

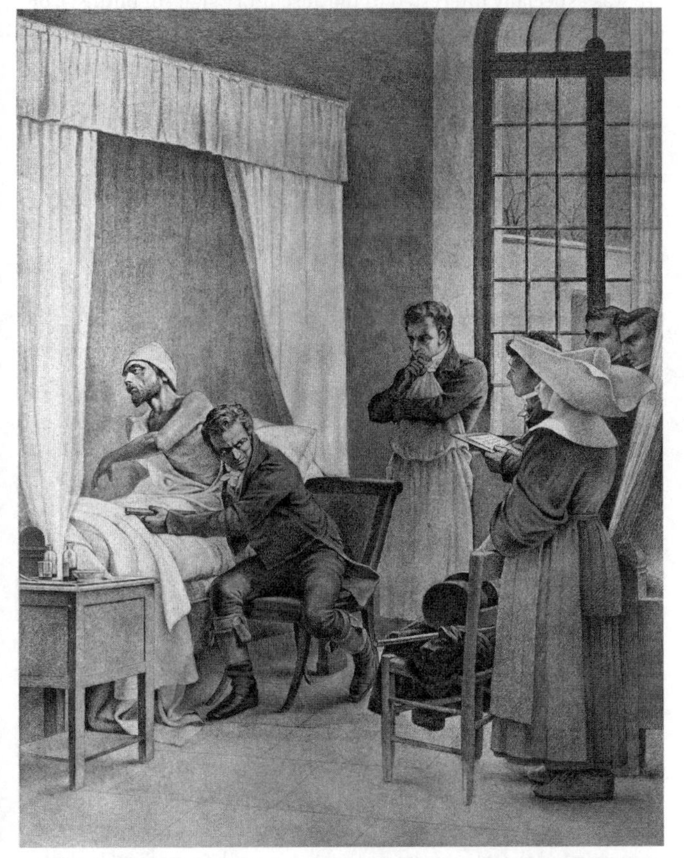

11. The late 19th-century reconstruction of Laennec demonstrating his stethoscope captures a bedside scene in a ward at the Necker Hospital. The patient is passive and extremely cachectic, suggestive of phthisis

in the whole history of medicine. By the time he published his treatise on mediate auscultation in the latter year, he was an accomplished stethoscopist. He created much of the vocabulary that doctors still use to describe breath sounds and argued cogently that he could diagnose many diseases of the heart and lungs by the specific auditory patterns revealed by his stethoscope. He was especially interested in the auscultory signs of phthisis, or consumption, the leading killer of Laennec's era. His wards were filled with its victims, and the disease eventually claimed him as another one.

Laennec's 1819 treatise consisted of two parts, one on the art of using the stethoscope, the other on the pathological anatomy of the organs of the thorax. He was a true disciple of the French school, versed not only in the nuances of diagnosis, but also routinely following his deceased patients from their bedside to the morgue, where he conducted the autopsy and compared the findings he had diagnosed in life with the lesions that were in the dead body.

Inspection, palpation, percussion, auscultation: these four steps in systematic medical examination were not adopted instantaneously and universally. More than a decade separates Corvisart's translation of Auenbrugger (1806) and Laennec's treatise on his stethoscope (1819). Laennec taught stethoscopy to a number of French and foreign students, and the value of his diagnostic instrument was recognized by a group of influential physicians. His English translator affirmed that private patients would not willingly submit to the intimacy of a stethoscopic examination, but it would be useful in 'captive' populations, that is, poor people in hospitals and military personnel. In fact, the power that doctors acquired in hospitals only gradually permeated outwards. He who pays the piper has ever called the tune, and paying patients had to be convinced that doctor knows best. A complete medical history and examination of the kind that French hospital doctors initiated is still a rare event outside of hospitals and diagnostic clinics. Nevertheless, the ideal elaborated by French clinicians in the Paris medical school still resonates and ought to be part of the mindset that doctors bring to the bedside.

To the morgue: clinico-pathological correlation

The Paris medical school was reopened with its reformed curriculum in 1794. Arguably, it was rooted earlier, in 1761. Auenbrugger's description of percussion appeared that year; so did Giovanni Battista Morgagni's *De sedibus et causis morborum* (On the Seats and Causes of Diseases), a work that underpinned the French pathological approach, just as Auenbrugger's little book contributed to its clinical one.

Morgagni's massive treatise was more an encyclopaedia than a textbook, organized in the traditional way of head-to-foot presentation. It offered case histories and autopsies of some 700 patients, many of them his own. Beginning with diseases of the head and working his way through the human body, Morgagni focused on the pathological changes that occur in the organs in disease. His case histories relied on the patient's own account of their illness, in ways that would have been familiar to the Hippocratics, and they also share the concern with close attention to detail. In addition, Morgagni brought that same case to the autopsy room, and his descriptions of morbid changes went well beyond the ancients, who of course performed no post-mortem examinations. Morgagni's work contains a number of original observations, but it was its method that reverberated. It was translated into most European languages and stimulated the use of the autopsy to learn about disease before the French school routinized it.

Morgagni (1682–1771) taught both anatomy and medicine at the University of Padua for more than 50 years. Many of the patients whose cases he included in *De sedibus* came from his extensive private practice, and although Morgagni's series of autopsies was impressive, it was soon dwarfed by the Paris school, whose clinicians practically lived in the hospitals and could accumulate in a couple of years as many post-mortem records as Morgagni collected during his long life. Hospitals offered concentrations of diseased humanity and the French exploited the conditions to the hilt.

If physical diagnoses helped the doctor find the lesion, the autopsy enabled him to interpret his earlier diagnoses and modify or reinforce them. Clinico-pathological correlation was thus a two-way street, with the repeated bedside observations giving the opportunity of following the patient's illness during his or her life, and these records being discussed in the light of the final observations on the corpse. The clinician was his own pathologist, caring for his patients in death as in life. Thus, Corvisart, Laennec, and the other leaders of the French school were equally at home at the bedside and the morgue.

They were driven by the search for the lesion, those pathological changes produced by disease. The philosopher Francis Bacon (1561–1626) called these changes 'the footsteps of disease', and the image is apposite, of some personified 'disease' walking through the organs of our bodies, leaving behind traces of its visit. Identifying these traces was the point of the post-mortem examination.

Post-mortems were conducted by French clinicians in the same spirit as the physical examination: to objectify the phenomena of disease, and thereby replace the speculations of 2,000 years with the hard, palpable, visible, weighable, material consequences of pathology. 'Open a few corpses', Xavier Bichat (1771–1802) had exclaimed, and the airy theories of the ancients would disappear. He himself opened more than just a few in his short life (he was 31 when he died), displaying nevertheless the perfect trajectory for what Paris medicine was all about. He had served in the military, and was a surgeon turned physician, thereby living that integration of the localist thinking of surgery with the more philosophical, thoughtful perspective of the physician. His death was widely mourned, and he quickly became a hero of the new medical ways of thinking.

He is remembered today mostly as the 'father of histology', since he recognized that pathological processes are common in the same kinds of tissue wherever they occur. Thus the serous membranes that line the heart, brain, thorax, and abdomen react in similar ways to disease processes. Working with the naked eye and a simple hand lens, he identified 21 such types of tissue, such as osseous, nervous, fibrous, or mucous. He also considered veins and arteries as special 'tissues'. Bichat was more intrigued by process than many of the French clinicians who were inspired by him, and brought a more theoretical perspective to his work than the flat-footed empiricism that characterized much of French hospital medicine. But he lived and died in the hospital, dividing his time between the bedside and dead room, and he inspired others both by his ideas and his energy, the latter extinguished too soon.

The hospitals of Paris (there were far more beds there than in the whole of Great Britain) offered an unparalleled opportunity to observe desperately sick people, drawn from the needy classes and required to offer their bodies, in life and in death, to the service of clinical medicine, in return for whatever care was on offer. The French combination of physical diagnoses and clinico-pathological correlation constituted a new approach to disease, and embodied new power structures within the hospital. It gradually produced a new organization (nosology) of disease, grounded in the organs, and elevating the solid parts of the body to pole position. It was arguably the Hippocratic approach writ large, but based in the hospital and situating disease in the organs rather than the humours.

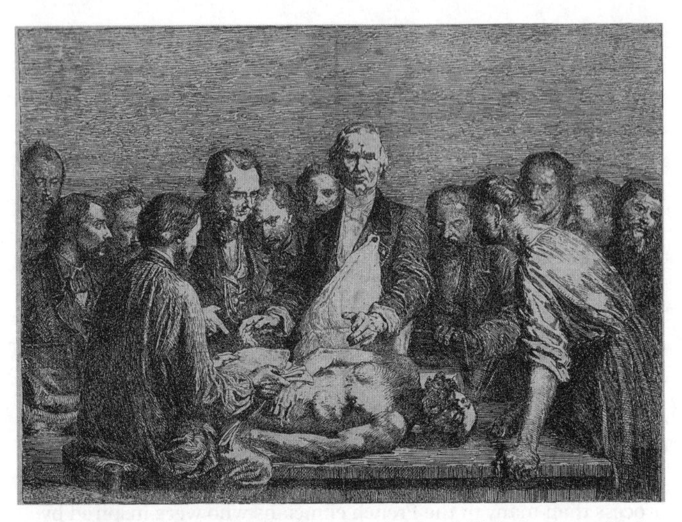

12. Alfred Velpeau (1795–1867) was professor of clinical surgery in the Paris Medical Faculty, but he also made contributions to surgical anatomy, embryology, physiology, and diseases of the breast. This sombre etching poignantly commemorates the uses of the dead for the living

Organ pathology became the dominant theme. Monographs on the diseases of the heart, lungs, kidneys, brain and nervous system, stomach and intestines, liver, skin, and reproductive organs became the way French clinicians made names for themselves. Corvisart's monograph on diseases of the heart and Laennec's on diseases of the lungs were linked to their diagnostic innovations. Others – Alibert on the skin, Rayer on the kidneys, Andral on the blood, Ricord on the reproductive organs – extended the approach to other parts of the body.

Of all diseases, phthisis was undoubtedly the most written about, and most commonly encountered among the patients (and their doctors) in the French hospitals. It was the leading cause of death throughout Europe in the early 19th century. 'Phthisis' (consumption) was described by the Hippocratics as a dangerous wasting disease with fever, chronic cough, and other pulmonary symptoms, and there is good palaeopathological evidence that tuberculosis has been common in human societies for millennia. Phthisis became ubiquitous from the late 18th century, and there is reason to suppose that most cases of 'phthisis' would today be diagnosed as tuberculosis. The latter disease category received its modern definition only when Robert Koch identified the bacterium, the tubercle bacillus, as the causative agent of tuberculosis in 1882. Nevertheless, Laennec and his colleagues defined 'phthisis' pathologically, and their descriptions of both the clinical symptoms and the post-mortem findings confirm the assumption that phthisis and tuberculosis are for the most part two names for the same disease.

Laennec claimed to be able to diagnose phthisis with his stethoscope, arguing for 'pathognomonic' (i.e. unique to that condition) sounds in the upper chest in patients with the affliction. He argued on both clinical and post-mortem grounds that the tiny lesion called the 'tubercle' (literally, a small swelling) was the hallmark of a single disease, no matter where the lesion was found. He thus unified a number of different diagnoses, such as scrofula, tuberculous meningitis, or tubercles of the intestine. He likened the development of larger granular lesions from the initial tubercles to the ripening of fruit. His grouping diseases of many organs containing tubercles into a single entity was vindicated by Koch's work on the bacillus, but within the pathological tradition, it took a leap of the imagination and was counter-intuitive given the organ-based paradigm within which he worked. As for the cause of phthisis, Laennec suspected that it would never be known for certain, although his own causative framework veered towards the psychosomatic. Strong passions were often associated with the disease, and he quietly assigned them causative significance.

Laennec's brilliant diagnostic work underscores both the strengths and weaknesses of the clinico-pathological approach: by concentrating on the end-stage of disease, the lesions, French clinicians were often left short on both the processes by which the lesions were formed, and the aetiology (cause) of the changes. More positively, by looking closely at the correlations between clinical signs and pathological changes, they were able to differentiate many diseases that have remained in the medical vocabulary, even after germ theory and other later developments offered different sets of diagnostic criteria.

One good example was the separation of typhus and typhoid fevers. The two words are similar and their clinical presentations could be close enough that it is sometimes difficult in the older medical literature to sort out one from the other, or from alternative conditions that might be diagnosed today. They were two varieties of fever, a disease in its own right in earlier times. In the 18th-century disease classifications, 'fever' was the disease, broken up into various kinds with adjectives such as intermittent, continued, typhus, typhoid, low, nervous, putrid, hectic. 'Typhoid fever' still sounds acceptable to us, and 'yellow fever' is the full name we use for the disease caused by a virus. These names linger even after 19th-century doctors gradually came to define 'fever' as a sign of disease (elevated body temperature, measured by a thermometer), rather than a disease itself.

The differentiation of typhus and typhoid was effected more or less independently by several doctors, each under the spell of the French way of doing medicine, but working in Britain and the United States as well as France. In France, Pierre Louis (1787–1872) established pathological criteria for typhoid in 1829. His career epitomizes the French era. Young enough to train in the 'new' medicine, he spent a few years in Russia before returning to Paris in 1820, convinced that he did not know enough about disease. He gave up private practice and attached himself to the Charité hospital, carrying out more than 2,000 autopsies over a six-year period and keeping elaborate records of both clinical and pathological findings. These became the basis of his subsequent monographs on phthisis and enteric fever (typhoid). Louis identified the swollen lymph nodes (Peyer's patches) in the membrane of the large intestine, arguing that they are pathognomonic for enteric fever. William Jenner (1815–98) in London, W. W. Gerhard (1809–72) in Philadelphia, and several others completed the differentiation of the two diseases.

During the first half of the 19th century, pathological anatomy was the queen of the medical sciences. It provided doctors with palpable evidence of the consequences of disease, which led to a streamlining of the elaborate nosologies of earlier times. It would not have been possible without the vast collections of patients in hospitals, allowing doctors to make clinical and pathological observations on so much 'material', as they often disparagingly called it. The numbers game constituted the third pillar, called by Louis, its most systematic practitioner, the *méthode numérique* (numerical method). He applied it to help gather his pictures of diagnostic categories, but also to evaluate therapy.

Learning to count

Like so much else in the Parisian hospitals, dealing with large numbers of patients was not entirely new to medicine. Military doctors of all nationalities had been pressed to provide statistics, and the doctors in hospitals, both military and civilian, had recognized the duty of presenting annual summaries of cases, diagnoses, treatments, and cures. One might view Louis as simply the culmination of the Enlightenment emphasis on facts and openness. This mistakes innovation for impact: of the later clinicians in the heyday of Paris medicine, Louis had the greatest international impact. He taught many foreign students and, more than any other, brought the insights of the French school together. His short essay on *Clinical Instruction*, translated into English in 1834, is a brilliant summary of what teaching and learning in Paris strove to be.

He is sometimes credited with almost single-handedly convincing doctors to abandon the ancient practice of bloodletting for all manner of diseases. His short monograph on the subject (1835) remains his best-known work, but its legacy lies more with the method than the message. In *Researches on the Effects of Bloodletting in Some Inflammatory Diseases*, Louis evaluated the effect of different timing (early or late) and quantity (a little or more vigorous) of therapeutic phlebotomy in cases of pneumonia. The same monograph also examined the use of different doses of tartar emetic (a medicine containing antimony). What is remembered today is the way Louis attempted to evaluate these therapies by dividing similar patients into groups and comparing the results of his various treatments. In effect, Louis was using a clinical trial, though hardly with a protocol that would now be judged adequate. Notice that Louis did not include *no* bloodletting as an option, but merely evaluated timing and quantity.

Louis' little monograph, despite its classic status, was actually part of a polemical campaign between Louis and F. J. V. Broussais (1772–1838). The latter had developed a system of 'physiological medicine' to counter the static, anatomical approach of most French clinicians. Broussais had noticed how many of the patients that he autopsied showed signs of chronic gastric irritation and his system posited that all disease originated in the stomach, and that local lesions elsewhere resulted from the primary irritation within the stomach. The standard treatment for irritation or inflammation was bloodletting. He favoured leeches rather than the lancet, and he and Louis exchanged a series of sharp polemics during the 1830s. Broussais was a therapeutic enthusiast, whereas Louis was quietly pessimistic about the capacity of medicine to do much to arrest the progress of disease. Louis's role as a pioneer of clinical trials was located within this ongoing feud with his rival Broussais.

Although Broussais' dynamic, physiological notions of disease continued to resonate, his central idea of all disease as a secondary consequence of gastric irritation did not long survive. On the other hand, Louis's numerical method has become essential to modern medicine. There was certainty in numbers, both in establishing clear diagnostic categories and in evaluating therapy. A number of his students assimilated his therapeutic scepticism, already common in the Paris hospitals where doctors were most concerned with accurate diagnosis and its verification through the post-mortem. Patients had almost always entered hospitals with limited expectations, but the power relationships shifted in Paris, with doctors on top. They remained that way until recently, when greater patient autonomy, the tyranny of economics, and the rise of the medical manager have realigned power structures within medicine.

Louis's recognition that he did not have much to offer his patients with the drugs at his disposal must be viewed not as a conspiracy against his helpless patients, but as a genuine discovery. It was made possible because he counted, evaluated, and compared: activities that could be done most easily in the hospital.

The physical and the mental

By 1850 or so, French hospital medicine had become familiar. New approaches to understanding disease, the greater use of experiment rather than mere observation, and diminishing returns on what could be discovered by yet one more autopsy, rendered the miracle of French clinical medicine something more pedestrian. During its heyday, however, thousands of students had come to Paris from all over the Western world. They returned to Britain, Germany, Austria, Italy, the United States, and the Netherlands, where some of them founded medical schools and hospitals. By the early 19th century, a medical school without an attached hospital was second rate. When the new University of London (now University College London) began its medical school in the late 1820s, the first thing to do was to establish a hospital. The pattern was repeated throughout Europe, even in small

German towns where clinical instruction was often by demonstration, not by doing.

In mid-century America, a number of proprietary schools prospered without a hospital or laboratory, offering medical degrees in return for a few months' tuition fees. Although returning students from Paris and graduates from the established East Coast medical schools, such as the University of Pennsylvania, despaired of what this did to the profession, American values protected entrepreneurialism. Only in the later decades of the century was the pattern broken. The Johns Hopkins University, established as a research-orientated university in 1876, introduced the German model of higher education to America. Despite a generous initial endowment by Johns Hopkins, a Quaker railway magnate, the medical school took almost two decades to be realized, so extensive were the requirements. The hospital opened in 1893, with the energetic faculty introducing a combination of German research and French emphasis on practical training. The professor of medicine, William Osler (1849–1919), was the most famous of the 'Big Four' – the initial senior medical faculty. He still commands adulation from doctors, as a scientifically attuned but humane clinician, book collector, historian, essayist, and teacher. The assimilation of German science infused the Hopkins approach to disease, but French innovations permanently left teaching hospitals with two regular events: the daily ward round, in which a senior clinician, followed by junior doctors, medical students, and a nurse, would see and discuss each patient at his or her bedside; and grand rounds, in which interesting 'cases' would be presented by a member of the junior staff and analysed by someone from the senior hierarchy, in front of a large gathering of students and doctors at all levels of experience. Often, after the presentation of the patient's history and clinical course, and the discussion of the differential diagnosis, the autopsy findings would be revealed by a pathologist, and the whole life and death of the patient put together in a seamless whole.

In the large teaching hospitals, the medical and surgical specialties, such as paediatrics, cardiology, neurology, obstetrics, orthopaedic surgery, or otolaryngology (diseases of the ear, nose, and throat), would each have their own chief, a number of dedicated beds, and regular rounds, both ward and grand. One speciality long under-represented in most general hospitals was psychiatry, even if psychiatry has been called 'half of medicine', so common are psychiatric disorders. Instead, those suffering from serious psychiatric illness – earlier called madness or lunacy – had their own kind of institutional setting. The institutional provision for the mad developed independently from the scattered provision of ordinary hospitals in the early-modern period. Madhouses, as they were brutally called, were usually small establishments, for profit, and as often as not run by a non-medical person. Unlike general hospitals, they were mostly for the well-to-do, so embarrassing was the behaviour of a seriously eccentric or hallucination-prone relative. The most famous psychiatric institution in Britain gave its name to the language: Bedlam, a short form of its full name, Bethlehem, or St Mary Bethlehem. 'Tom-o-Bedlam' became a stock fictional character, used by Shakespeare in King Lear, and symptomatic of the isolation that psychiatric patients have always felt.

Bedlam was unusual among psychiatric institutions, funded by endowments and with governors overseeing its operations. Most madhouses were small private affairs whose records have long since disappeared from view. But they entered public consciousness, since madness was the most feared disorder of earlier centuries (dementia often occupies that place now, even more than cancer for many people). Madhouses, not usually dignified by the name 'hospital', occupied the opposite end of the scale from ordinary hospitals. Diagnosis relied on what the neighbours or family reported, or observations about the patient's behaviour. Doctors who looked for lesions, the basis of Paris medicine, were usually disappointed. The brains of lunatics rarely pointed to some specific reason why the patient displayed symptoms. Madness was mental, not physical, even if that posed difficulties for a culture which assumed that the distinctly human characteristics of reason, moral responsibility, and the capacity to know right from wrong were the consequences of our immortal, God-given souls. Loss of reason meant loss of humanity.

These philosophical and theological niceties were negotiated in various ways, but as doctors became increasingly involved in the 'trade in lunacy', the disease model became more attractive. After all, disease is what doctors deal with. Fittingly, one of the father-figures of Parisian medicine is often called the founder of modern psychiatry. Philippe Pinel (1745–1826) made his name before the Revolution, as the author of a successful nosology of all diseases (he coined the word 'neurosis') and a medical practitioner. He also wrote a little treatise on the importance of hospitals for clinical instruction. During the Revolution, he was given the post of physician to the Bicêtre (male), and then the Salpêtrière (female), each a large *Hôpital Général* which housed a variety of inmates. These included prostitutes, vagabonds, petty criminals, orphans, the aged, decrepit, and demented, as well as other individuals deemed a danger to the wider public or unable to fend for themselves in society at large. The Revolution turned these institutions into hospitals for psychiatric patients, and during his tenure at the Salpêtrière, Pinel gradually instituted a programme of 'moral therapy', slowly releasing confined women and treating them with firm humanity. In England, a Quaker family, the Tukes, founded the York Retreat. It was based on similar therapeutic principles of moral therapy, which were also employed at roughly the same time in Italy, by Vincenzio Chiarugi (1759–1820).

The nuances of moral therapy have been much debated by historians, but there is little doubt that this form of treatment brought the lunatic into the public gaze, and helped create a psychiatric specialty within medicine. During the middle third of the 19th century, psychiatric associations were established in most

European countries and the United States, and they successfully campaigned for the establishment of networks of psychiatric hospitals (generally called 'asylums'). The traditional treatment of psychiatric disorders with ordinary medicaments –bloodletting, emetics, cathartics – was replaced by 'moral' means, and the actual form of the buildings was held to aid in the healing process. From the 1830s, non-restraint became the rallying cry, as doctors argued that the well-designed and well-run psychiatric institution had no need to use physical restraint with its patients.

Although the asylums were built in the name of humanity and treatment, they hardly justified the early optimism, by which early diagnoses and the expert use of moral and other therapies were predicted to produce cures. Instead, the asylums grew larger and silted up with incurable patients; they became, in the words of one contemporary commentator, mere 'museums of madness'. The special nature of these institutions reinforced the distance between psychiatry and ordinary medicine and surgery, a breach that still exists, despite modern knowledge of the brain and how it functions.

In the late 19th century, the German psychiatrist Emil Kraepelin (1856–1926) attempted to bring medicine and psychiatry closer together, through a psychiatric clinic within an academic setting. Kraepelin, an almost exact contemporary of the founder of psychoanalysis, Sigmund Freud (1856–1939), developed the broad classification of psychiatric disorders that formed the basis of modern psychiatric nosology. He differentiated the major psychoses from the neuroses, and provided a fundamental characterization of what is now called schizophrenia. Kraepelin called it dementia praecox, the dementia of younger people, and his efforts helped to create academic psychiatry.

The gap between medicine and psychiatry still exists, but the trajectory of the discipline from asylum to clinic highlights the

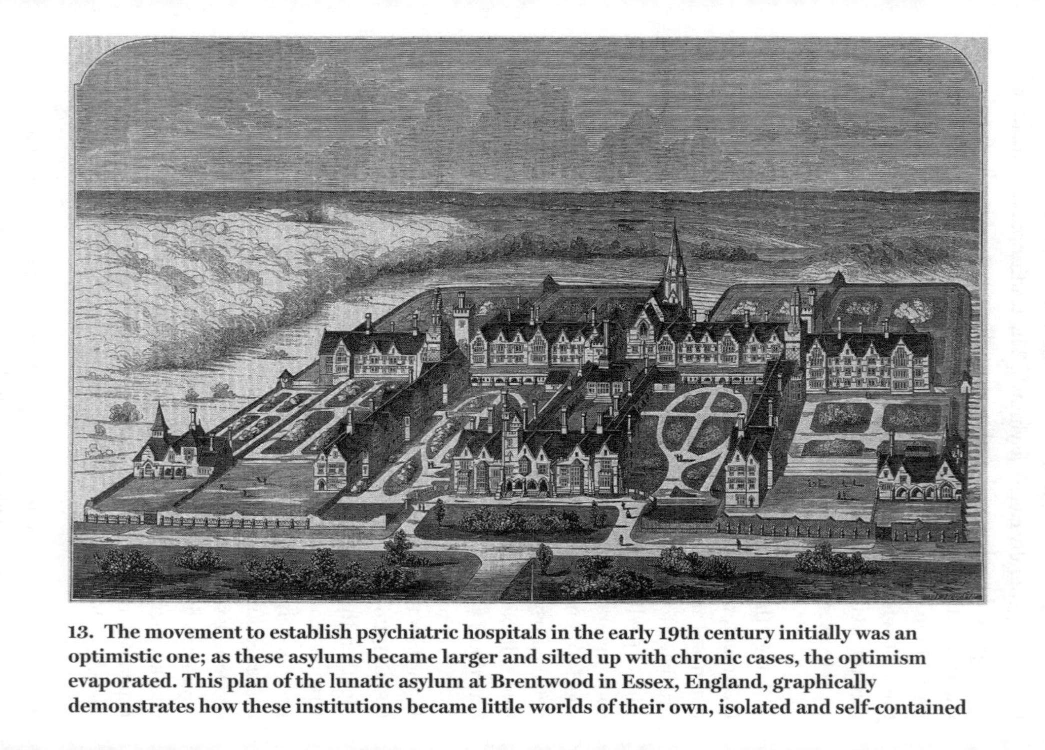

13. The movement to establish psychiatric hospitals in the early 19th century initially was an optimistic one; as these asylums became larger and silted up with chronic cases, the optimism evaporated. This plan of the lunatic asylum at Brentwood in Essex, England, graphically demonstrates how these institutions became little worlds of their own, isolated and self-contained

faith that Western societies have put in hospitals as healing institutions, as well as the increasing medicalization of many aspects of living, from sadness to criminality, from rebellious behaviour to attention deficit disorder syndrome. Putting a name on something is in itself comforting, and Kraepelin sought to impose a diagnostic order on mental disturbances just as the French clinicians had earlier used physical diagnosis to understand the diseases of our bodies.

Chapter 4
Medicine in the community

The people's health

The modern public health movement began in the 19th century. It was built, of course, on earlier political, social, and medical structures, but the form in which we know it emerged only a couple of centuries ago. If the relationship between patients and their doctors situates hospital medicine, public health is about the state and the individual. It is at once the most anonymous part of medicine and the most visible. When we go to the hospital, not many people notice. When there is an outbreak of influenza, or the water supply is contaminated, it is newsworthy.

As the name implies, public health is concerned with maintaining health and preventing or containing disease. Its traditional brief was with epidemic disease, but there was always another strand of disease prevention, aimed at preserving the health of the individual, and termed hygiene. Although these represent two different traditions within medicine, they are often intertwined, sharing the object of preventing disease. Increasingly, hygiene has been collapsed into the phrase 'lifestyle medicine'. In both strands, the state plays a crucial role.

Before the industrial state

There are many references to epidemic diseases in ancient literature. Indeed, before modern times, human populations were periodically thinned by the Malthusian horsemen of the apocalypse, subsistence crises and disease. Much life was nasty, brutish, and short. In the long history of the Malthusian pressures of destitution and disease, the plague years, from the mid-14th to the mid-17th centuries, stand out as particularly grim.

The Black Death, as the Victorians called it, was arguably the first pandemic (intercontinental or worldwide epidemic) in history. Most earlier plagues were more confined in space, and generally also in time. The Black Death took more than four years to make its way via the Silk Road from the Steppes of Central Asia to the westernmost parts of Europe, the Middle East, and the northern shores of Africa. It wiped out between one quarter and one half of the population of Europe, and was the first of a series of devastating epidemics that lost its Western European hold only in the 1660s (an outbreak in the 1720s in Marseilles was contained).

It is certain that the Black Death was *a* plague, since that word refers to any highly virulent epidemic. It has recently become fashionable to argue that the plague of the 1340s was not caused by the plague bacillus, *Yersinia pestis*, identified in Hong Kong during the last pandemic in the 1890s. Various other organisms have been suggested, since the Black Death had some features that do not conform to what we know about the epidemiology of modern bubonic plague. Its rate of spread, seasonality, and mortality patterns, together with the fact that nobody noticed a lot of dead rats (modern human plague outbreaks are accompanied with rat or other rodent plagues), have led some commentators to postulate that anthrax, an unknown virus, or other infectious agent was the actual cause. Ergot poisoning has also been invoked.

The problem with these alternative interpretations is that they concentrate almost exclusively on the original pandemic, the Black Death. If one looks at the plague years as a whole, from 1345 to 1666, the pattern is more certain. By the later years, the plague (for instance, the Great Plague of London in 1665) is more easily recognizable through medical and other accounts. Furthermore, the disease was perceived by those who lived through the various

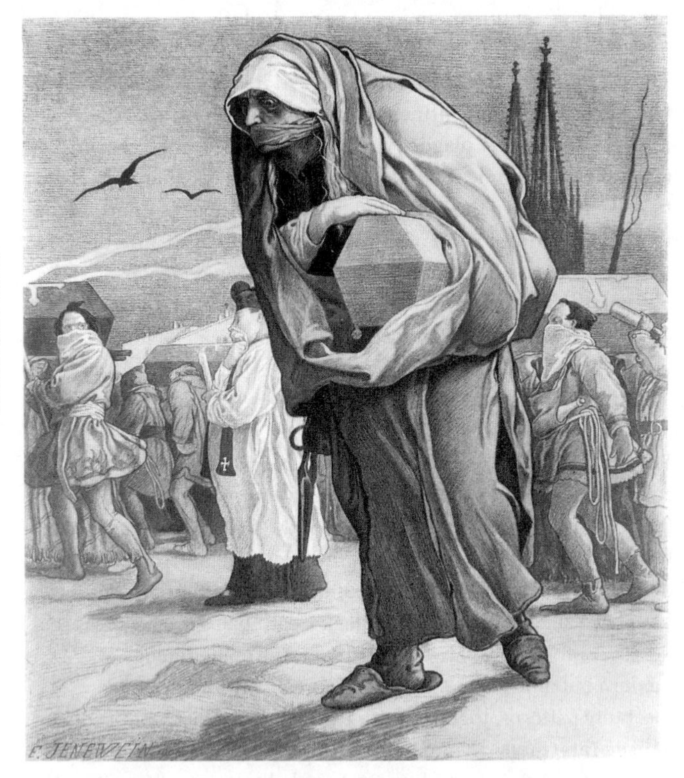

14. This modern lithograph by Felix Jenewein captures the desolation and panic that the repeated epidemics of bubonic plague created during the late Middle Ages and early-modern period. Our own fears of influenza or a terrorist-induced pandemic of smallpox or anthrax maintain the power of such images

epidemics as a single entity, and while of course no one experienced them all, there were always doctors who had lived through the previous epidemic or two. The collective historical experience is of a single, repeated disease, almost certainly 'our' plague; that is, the disease caused by the plague bacillus. The first epidemic attacked a population with no previous immunological experience, and there are many instances of such devastating outbreaks of other diseases (for instance, smallpox and measles) in virgin populations.

The range of causes put forward at the time ranged from the wrath of God to human sinfulness and sloth, marginal human groups such as Jews and witches, to bad air. Astrological causes were also frequently invoked. Despite the range of supernatural explanations on offer, the repeated plague epidemics also heightened awareness of communal health issues and called out a number of measures designed to prevent or contain the disease. Isolation, enforced border controls, compulsory hospitalization, and other measures aimed at the individual who might be afflicted were combined with more general measures such as routine quarantine of ships coming from plague areas, control of the movement of persons and goods, and medical inspection. The disease tested the limits of early-modern public health activity and demonstrates the inevitable nexus of the state and medicine during such times of crisis. Some historical scholarship has suggested that the *cordon sanitaire* along the southern and eastern edges of the Austro-Hungarian Empire might have had some effect in limiting the introduction of plague from the Middle East, where it remained endemic, and periodically epidemic, long after it disappeared from Western Europe; 19th-century European travellers in the area accepted the possibility of quarantine in one of the lazarettos maintained for control of its spread.

At the very least, plague ensured that issues of communal health and disease remained. The extent to which it led to any permanent public health infrastructure is debatable, although plague hospitals were built throughout Europe, and these were often used for isolating and treating other infectious diseases after plague disappeared. In general, the absolutist states of Europe developed some formal public health activities as part of the bureaucratic tentacles of the state. From the late 17th century, the notion of 'medical police' was developed in the German-speaking states. It reached its apogee with the nine-volume *System der vollständigen medicinischen Polizey* (1779–1827) by Johann Peter Frank (1745–1821), the cosmopolitan physician and public health reformer. The German word '*Polizey/Polizei*' is usually translated as 'police' in English, and Frank believed that formidable powers should be given to this department of government. His massive work dealt with virtually the whole of life, from cradle to grave: maternal, infant, and child care, dress, housing, paving, lighting, and the disposal of the dead. We are hardly the first to realize how much of human life has a direct bearing on health.

Frank's latter volumes appeared posthumously, and the set extended over the time when vaccination (which Frank enthusiastically espoused) began systematically to replace inoculation, as a specific preventative against smallpox. These two measures were the first specific preventatives, and although both were adopted by doctors, their origins were in folk medicine. Inoculation (the English word was taken from horticulture, and roughly is equivalent to grafting) involved the introduction of material taken from a pustule of someone suffering from smallpox, and introducing it into the body of someone who had not had the disease. It made sense on two counts. First, smallpox was a virtually universal disease, with a significant mortality, ranging according to circumstances between 5% and 20%. The analogy with chickenpox parties, where parents seek to expose their children to another child with the disease, to get it over with, is only partially apposite, since inoculation carried a significant risk, but the strategy was the same, even if the stakes were higher. Second, it was recognized that a single episode of the disease conferred life-long immunity, and by selecting a mild case to obtain the material for inoculation, the life-long chances of dying from the disease were reduced.

Inoculation was an ancient Eastern procedure. The Chinese practised it, using a powder of the pox material and taking it like snuff. In Turkey, the material was introduced through a scratch in the skin, and it was this technique that Lady Wortley Montague (1689–1762) learned about when she was in Constantinople as the wife of the British ambassador. She had her children, who had not had smallpox, inoculated, and they acquired mild cases of the disease. She and the physician to the British Embassy both made this innovation known in London, where it was taken up, after the monarch, George II, had his own children inoculated by the royal surgeon. James Jurin, a prominent London physician and disciple of Isaac Newton, collected statistics from a number of inoculators and showed mathematically that the chances of dying from the disease were significantly diminished by the practice.

By the mid-18th century, inoculation had been simplified and became more widespread, especially after the King of France, Louis XV, died of smallpox and his son, the ill-fated Louis XVI, was successfully inoculated in 1774. The procedure was never without difficulties, however, since patients sometimes died of the disease after being inoculated, and in any case, they became possible sources of spread to others.

Like many other general practitioners, Edward Jenner (1749–1823) occasionally inoculated his patients. In the Gloucestershire countryside near his practice, it was known that an occasional affliction of cattle, cowpox, sometimes produced what looked like a single pock on the hands of the milkmaids, and that they seemed protected from the more serious smallpox. Although a farmer named Jesty and other people had previously injected the cowpox material into individuals with the intent of preventing smallpox, Jenner performed the crucial experiment in

1796 and publicized the new preventative. He took some matter from a cowpox lesion on the hand of a milkmaid, Sarah Nelmes, and injected it into the arm of a young boy, James Phipps, who had not had natural smallpox. He developed a soreness and scab on his arm but, except for a day's fever, remained well. Six weeks later, Jenner inoculated him with ordinary smallpox material. He failed to develop the disease, showing that he was immune.

The Royal Society declined to publish his original paper, so in 1798 Jenner privately published his short treatise on the procedure he called 'vaccination', after the Latin word for cow. Unsurprisingly, the novel approach attracted some adverse comment, especially about the 'contamination' of human beings with animal material, and historians have puzzled about some of the outcomes of early vaccinations (some of the 'lymph', as the vaccinating material was called, may have been contaminated with ordinary smallpox matter). Nevertheless, Jenner's work was taken up quickly in Britain and abroad. He received two handsome grants from the British Parliament and could devote himself to furthering the vaccination cause.

'If preventable, why not prevented?', the future King Edward VII once asked of doctors. It was a good question, but the depressing answer is that it might cost too much, there might not be sufficient political or medical will, or that people (and their doctors) have to be educated about prevention, and education never takes universally. Although the smallpox story eventually ended as Jenner himself foresaw, with the eradication of the disease, in 1979, it was the exception rather than the rule. Prevention has ever been the poor relation of other forms of doctoring, despite the urgency of the case in industrializing societies.

Cholera and poverty: motors of public health

Historians traditionally viewed the 19th-century public health movement as a direct response to the series of cholera pandemics of the period. The first epidemic to reach Europe (the first pandemic of 1817–23 petered out after it spread from India to the Middle East and northern Africa) certainly raised consciousness about communal disease. From 1827, when the second pandemic began to spread out from its ordinary home in eastern India, Europe watched anxiously as the disease moved ever closer. Many European nations sent delegates at some stage during the four-year waiting game, to investigate the disease and make recommendations on how best to prevent its reaching Europe.

There were two main sources of concern. First, the disease was new to the West, an 'exotic' disease with which only tropical colonials would have had previous experience. The second pandemic moved throughout Europe and into North America, and introduced the medical profession to a serious new disorder with alarming symptoms and mortality rate. Its newness and epidemic character led many commentators to speak of the return of the plague, all the more disturbing since old-style bubonic plague seemed to have disappeared permanently from the West.

Second, the pattern of spread was puzzling. Two polarized explanatory paradigms were current to explain epidemic diseases: miasmatic and contagious. Miasmatists argued that communal diseases were spread through the air, the result of atmospheric conditions or particles contained in the air. The most commonly postulated source of the disease was rotting organic matter, such as refuse, faeces – anything, in fact, that was oppressive or smelled badly. The power of this paradigm is easily appreciated: the air is a common feature of a locality and could explain why many individuals might be affected. It also helped differentiate 'healthy' from 'unhealthy' localities, within a paradigm that would have been familiar to the author of the Hippocratic treatise *Airs, Waters, Places*. It was the dominant explanation for the complex of diseases, many of them unknown in the Old World, which Europeans encountered in tropical areas.

They were generally known simply as 'diseases of warm climates', and oppressive heat and humidity and exotic vegetation were so obvious that evoking them to explain disease patterns made rational sense.

Contagionists postulated that epidemic diseases were spread from one afflicted individual to another. This could account for many aspects of epidemic disease, such as the fact that people nursing sick individuals often came down with the disease themselves. Contagionism justified the instinctive wish to avoid contact with people suffering from dangerous diseases, and underlay the practice of quarantine. It also preyed on collective fears of the origin of plague and other frightful diseases in marginalized groups.

A middle position, 'contingent contagionism', was less hard-line, and more easily adaptable to the anomalies that both the main positions had difficulty explaining. Contingent contagionists argued that diseases might be either miasmatic or contagious, depending on the circumstances. For instance, a disease might enter the community through corrupt air but some individuals could develop the disease in such a way that they then became foci of contagious spread. This mixed the categories in ways that the observations required, and covered all fronts. Unfortunately, theories that explain everything often explain very little.

A few diseases, such as smallpox and measles, were always viewed as contagious, but most communicable diseases had patterns of incidence and spread that were sufficiently complicated to leave much room for debate. Germ theory was later to offer a new paradigm for communicable and epidemic diseases, although there were still anomalies: why could two people exposed to the same source of infection react in such different ways, so that one came down with the disease and the other remained completely well?

Before germ theory, there was little consensus, and in practice communities often covered both alternatives. In plague outbreaks, for instance, quarantine and isolation were accompanied with fires, to purify the air, and nosegays, infusing the immediate inhalations. When in doubt, do both.

Cholera threw up these age-old issues in an urgent manner. The observers who went to watch its westward march came back with mixed reactions. Some thought that it was contagious and Europe's best response was isolation and quarantine. Others believed that the air was the vehicle and that ordinary sanitary improvements – improving drainage, keeping the streets clean – were the best defence. European governments listened to the variety of opinions but mostly fell back on the time-honoured solution of quarantine and inspection of people and goods arriving from the infected areas.

Even Britain, home of *laissez-faire*, dabbled with quarantine during the first pandemic to reach Western Europe, from 1830. Cholera arrived in Britain in late 1831, in Sunderland, a port in the north-east, and then travelled gradually in all directions, reaching London in early 1832. Its pattern of spread convinced miasmatists that the air was the culprit, and contagionists that it was propagated by human beings. Almost everyone had to conclude, after the epidemic had played itself out, that the system of quarantine had not done its job. Thereafter, British policy relied primarily on port inspection and isolation of suspicious cases, covering both paradigms. Britain had then by far the largest maritime commitment, and therefore the most to lose by costly and disruptive employment of quarantine. A regular series of International Sanitary conferences were held from 1851, primarily concerned with cholera. Britain and British India stood firm together in opposing quarantine as a routine agent of disease control. The economic consequences of such a policy were clear to all, and Britain's scientific policy was blatantly dictated by commercial considerations.

The scent lies strong here; do you see any thing?
Positively we must find something; it wont do to lose our Twenty guineas a day
CHOLERA MORBUS
Oh! if I can but find a smell
Looseness of the bowels is the beginning of the Cholera
A LONDON BOARD OF HEALTH HUNTING AFTER CASES LIKE CHOLERA.

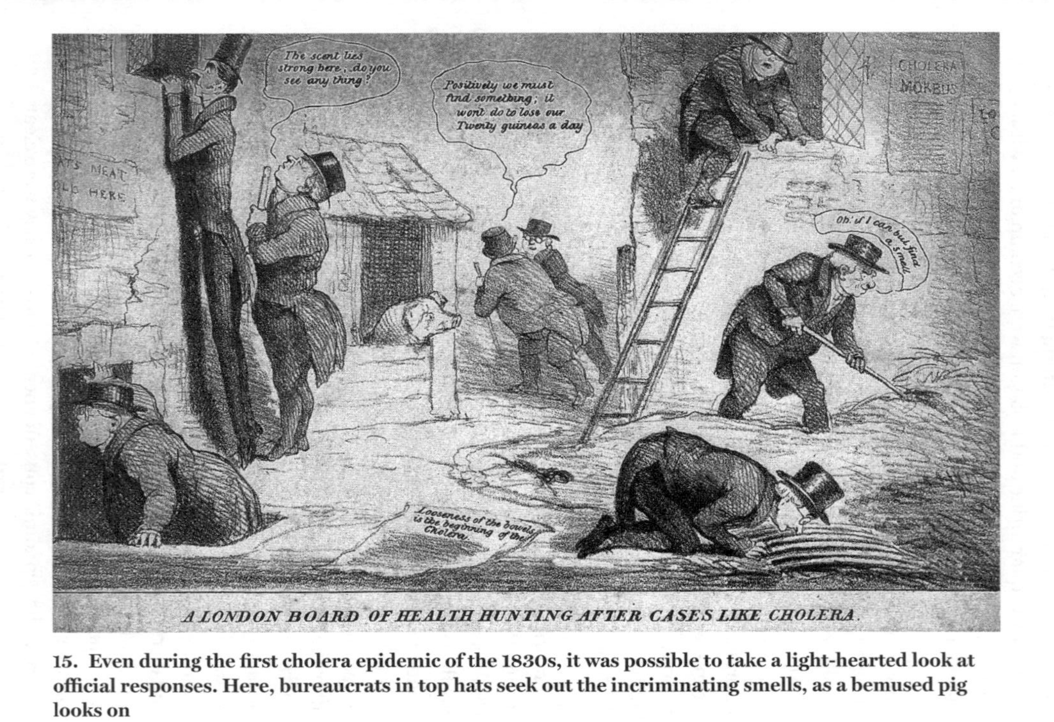

15. Even during the first cholera epidemic of the 1830s, it was possible to take a light-hearted look at official responses. Here, bureaucrats in top hats seek out the incriminating smells, as a bemused pig looks on

The miasmatic position was consolidated by the leading figure in the early British public health movement, Edwin Chadwick (1800–90). A lawyer by training, Chadwick had been the last secretary of the utilitarian philosopher and reformer Jeremy Bentham (1748–1832). From Bentham, Chadwick absorbed the doctrines of efficiency and the simple equation of good with happiness ('the greatest good for the greatest number' is the slogan of utilitarianism). Chadwick came to public health through his concern with poverty, and in particular the operation of the Poor Law, the legislative means of dealing with issues relating to the relief of poverty and destitution. The Old Poor Law, dating back to the late 16th century, had become woefully inadequate in a society undergoing rapid industrialization and urbanization. Britain was the first industrial nation, and the older ways of dealing with the poor were inappropriate in an industrial wage economy, with seasonal unemployment, urban poverty, and a growing class consciousness.

The brunt of the first European cholera epidemic was felt in 1832, an eventful year in other ways. A Reform Bill in Parliament went some way towards redressing unequal Parliamentary representation, the result of population shifts consequent on the rapid growth of industrial cities; the Bill also extended the franchise. Parliament set up a Poor Law Commission to examine how the Old Poor Law operated and make recommendations for its reform. This came after years of intense debate, part of it stimulated by T. R. Malthus's *Essay on the Principle of Population* (first edition, 1798; sixth edition, 1826). Malthus had pointed out the double-edged nature of poor relief: keeping the poor alive could simply compound the misery of penury in later generations, when breeding paupers reproduced yet more dependency. The 'law of population' that Malthus elaborated stated that throughout nature, the capacities of organisms to reproduce always outstripped the number of offspring that could actually survive. Human beings were not exempt from this stern law, with the

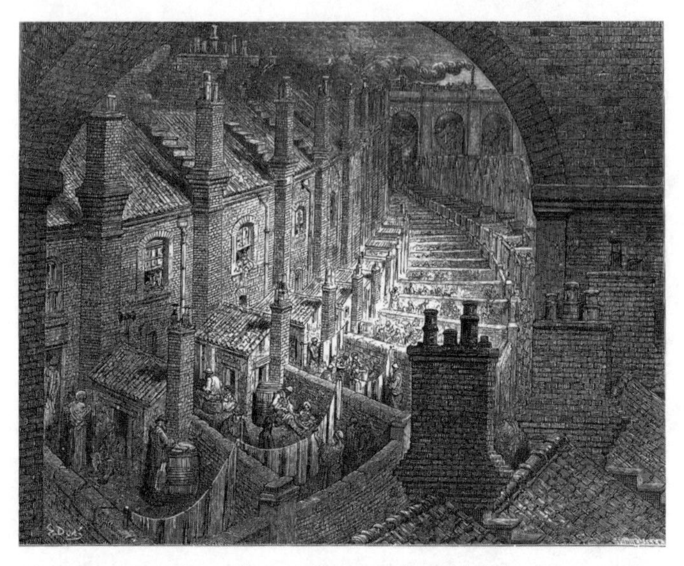

16. Gustave Dore's *London: A Pilgrimage* (1872) brilliantly captured the overcrowding and poverty of the largest and richest city in Europe

disparity caused by geometrical population increase set against the arithmetical increase in the means of subsistence. Disease, misery, war, vice, and want kept human populations down, and interfering with the system by keeping more pauper children alive did no good in the long run.

The Malthusian dilemma was merely one of the issues that the 1832 Poor Law Commission had to consider. Chadwick was its secretary and dominant figure, masterminding the systematic survey of how the 15,000 local parishes actually administered the Old Poor Law. Initiated in the time of Elizabeth I, in the late 16th century, this statute was designed to provide, from local taxes, a last safeguard for people who could not support themselves, through sickness, injury, unemployment, or other misfortunes. Designed for an overwhelmingly static, rural society, the Law had become increasingly inadequate, as Britain became more mobile, industrial, and urban, and reached a crisis after the close of the Napoleonic Wars in the 1810s, when thousands of military men returned home and could not find work. With 15,000 different local authorities administering it, there was wide disparity, something which deeply offended Chadwick's utilitarian leanings. The Commissioners' Report, published in 1834 and the basis for the New Poor Law of the same year, recommended streamlining and unifying its operations, so that similar rules and regulations extended over the whole country.

This New Poor Law, so hated by many for its harshness, served as the mechanism for poor relief until its abolition in 1929. Chadwick wanted to be a Commissioner of the new government department but had to content himself with being its paid Secretary. Administering the New Poor Law on a daily basis inevitably confronted Chadwick with the relationships between poverty and disease. Doctors had long noticed that epidemic diseases generally afflicted the poor more than the rich, and assumed that this was associated with their overcrowded living conditions, sparse diet, and other trappings of want. Chadwick's initial concern was with the fact that many of the demands on the Poor Law were because the breadwinner had fallen sick and could not work.

Disease could thus impoverish a family. The reverse proposition was more subtle: does poverty itself cause disease? Chadwick and many of his contemporaries preferred to put a moral spin on poverty *per se*, arguing that its ultimate cause lay in individual failing: imprudent marriages, failure to save, spending on drink and other vices. Nevertheless, since disease was a major factor in the causation of poverty, it followed that preventing what he called 'filth diseases' would ease the burden on the Poor Rate. As an ardent miasmatist, he attributed filth diseases such as cholera, typhus, and scarlet fever to the bad smells of rotting organic matter. The solution was easy: cleanliness. Dirt caused disease; cleanliness prevented it.

Chadwick's journey from a Poor Law reformer to one obsessed with preventing disease occurred over the few years from 1834 to 1842, when he published a classic text of the early public health movement: *Report on the Sanitary Condition of the Labouring Population of Great Britain*. He used the new statistical approaches of the day (the civil registration of births, marriages, and deaths had started in 1837) to quantify the staggering differences of mortality rates and average expectation of years at birth between overcrowded, urban areas and rural ones, and between the rich and the poor. To solve the problem of filth diseases, Chadwick proposed what he called an arterio-venous system of water supply and sewage disposal. If running water under pressure were supplied to households, cleanliness would be easier; if sewage were taken away in glazed pipes impervious to leakage, the problems of cesspits and ground contamination would be solved. Further, if the sewage were taken away from cities to treatment plants, it could be turned to guano, sold to farmers at a profit, and crops would be increased, thereby improving nutrition. It was a neat engineering solution to public health, good in its context, though not solving all the problems that Chadwick's limited view of disease causation envisioned.

He got his chance to influence public health in 1848, when cholera returned, and a Board of Health was established, with Chadwick one of three members (a fourth, a doctor, was added later). The Parliamentary Act setting up the Board was largely permissive, allowing communities to appoint a Medical Officer of Health (MoH) if 10% of their rate-payers petitioned for it. The MoH was obligatory only if the crude death rate in the area was greater than 23 per 1,000. The permissive clause was something of a Trojan Horse, since the MoHs raised the profile of prevention, and agitated for such officers throughout the country, on a statutory basis. This passage from permissive to statutory legislation became the pattern in liberal, *laissez-faire* societies, in ways that are still resonant. Investigating almost any social issue uncovers others that need attention.

Throughout his long life, Chadwick never abandoned his notion of filth disease, nor of the healing power of cleanliness. He left office against his will, in 1854, despite the return of cholera. His dictatorial style made too many enemies, and he wanted compulsory legislation to enter through the front door. It came, piecemeal and gradually, through the back one.

In the meantime, the nature of filth diseases was being reconceptualized. Only in hindsight did people realize that the Italian microscopist Filippo Pacini (1812–83) had described during the 1854 pandemic the causative organism of cholera. Of equal moment, the London anaesthetist, epidemiologist, and general practitioner John Snow (1813–58) demonstrated that cholera is not air but water borne. Snow was a medical apprentice during the original cholera outbreak in 1831–2, and studied the disease as an established and ambitious practitioner during the 1848 and 1854 London epidemics. He provided good evidence from the 1848 epidemic that the disease was transmitted through water contaminated by faeces; he nailed his case through two classic community experiments during 1854. The Broad Street Pump is the most famous – the stuff of legends. This pump, in Soho, central London (the street is now called Broadwick Street), served many houses, most of which had no direct access to running water. By systematically investigating house to house the cases that occurred in the area of a single water pump, and tracing cases further afield from people who had drunk water from the pump, he incriminated it as the source of the disease. An open sewer drained into it. The dramatic removal of the pump handle was more symbolic than effective, since the epidemic was already on the wane, but the incident attracted a good deal of attention.

His second epidemiological investigation was more impressive. He compared the incidence of people buying Thames water from two separate companies: one filtered their water and drew it upstream, before the sewers of London had emptied into it; the other used unfiltered water from downstream, sewerage and all. In some instances, people in the same streets, living in similar housing and breathing the same air, had contracts with each of the two companies. He showed that people using the water of the 'bad' company had 13 times the chance of coming down with cholera than people using the better supplies.

Snow's evidence seems obvious to us. It wasn't to most of his contemporaries, and the nature and cause of cholera continued to be debated for decades, even, it turns out, after Robert Koch described the organism in 1884, in an age of bacteriology. Old ways of thinking die hard, although when cholera struck Hamburg during the 1890s pandemic, more people listened to Koch than had to Snow four decades previously. His evidence was impressive, but so was Snow's. As the next chapter will show, only with the coming of science did real heroes emerge within modern medicine.

Establishing the public health bureaucracy

'In the beginning was the Word', St John's Gospel has it. Now, there is mostly the number. We live by the clock, follow the ups and downs of the stock markets or mortgage rates, experience the hottest, or wettest, month since records began. Contemporary society is permeated with numbers; they rule our lives.

Public health evidence is inevitably numerical. If the public health movement was in large measure a product of the industrialization and urbanization that transformed the Western world from the late 18th century, it also relied on the numerical mentality that accompanied the profits and losses of the factory system, the harnessing of steam, double-entry book-keeping, and the national census. Like us, the Victorians felt overwhelmed with facts and data.

Three dimensions to the quantification of medicine (and society more generally) should be highlighted: surveys, surveillance, and significance.

The survey is the most basic. The 1832 Poor Law Commission has been described as the pioneering national survey, and it certainly was novel for its times. Chadwick and his fellow commissioners sent out a detailed questionnaire to each of the parishes responsible for Poor Law relief, and attempted to coordinate the replies. In the late 1830s, Chadwick commissioned surveys of the relationship between poverty, overcrowding, and filth diseases. One of the first acts of Chadwick's successor as leader of the British Public Health Movement, John Simon (1816–1904), was a European-wide survey of vaccination and its effectiveness, in relation to the issue of enforcing compulsory vaccination. This survey convinced him that the way to prevent smallpox was to have an active policy of free vaccination. During his years in office, Simon gradually became disillusioned with persuasion as a tool to achieve public health ends, and under his leadership, Britain acquired a vaccination system that was publicly funded, free, universal, and compulsory, with penalties for non-compliance.

Throughout the developed world, during the middle decades of the 19th century, the power of the number became appreciated. Social issues with medical ramifications were repeatedly investigated by surveys. Issues of poverty, child labour, factory conditions, food adulteration, water supply, prostitution, building standards, and, of course, epidemic diseases, all came under scrutiny. Investigating one issue often threw up others that called out for attention. For instance, concern with the employment of young children in poorly paid and grinding jobs raised more general issues of education and child health. Charles Dickens's

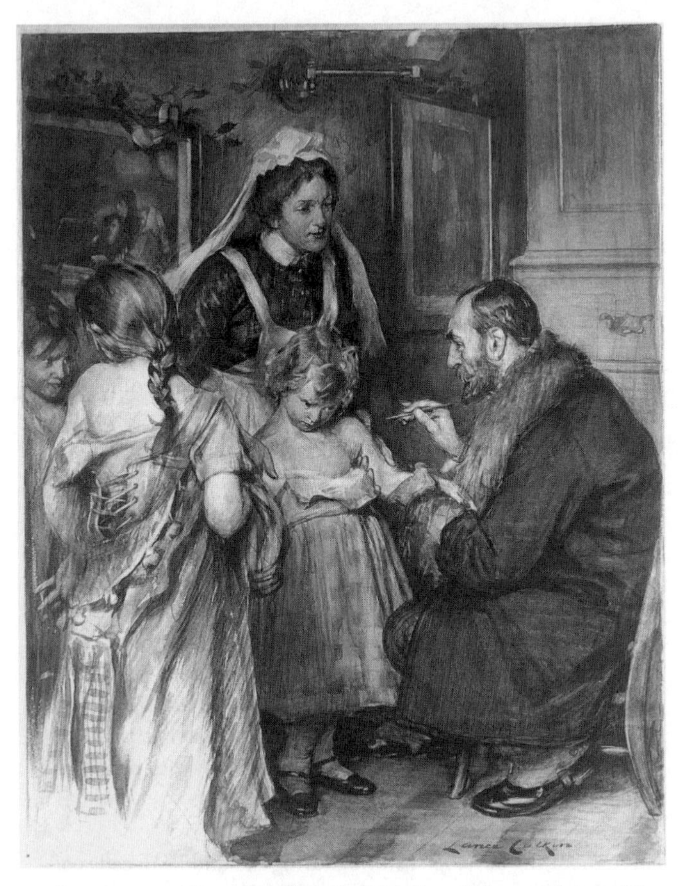

17. In contrast to Figure 15, when the intrusion of the state into public affairs is treated as an object of satire, here, in this image by Lance Calkin (c. 1901), the public vaccinator is seen as a figure of authority, quietly going about his work of protecting these young girls from smallpox

Mr Gradgrind was not the only one in 19th-century Europe who wanted 'the facts', and 'facts' increasingly came in a table or other quantitative form.

If surveys threw up all kinds of medical and social issues, surveillance was a complementary strategy, aimed at systematically following trends or following up on troubling problems. Many surveillance structures have long histories. For example, from medieval times, French butchers could expect periodic visits from inspectors examining the meat they were selling. Markets and fairs were conducted under regulations. Borders, ports, and walled towns were manned, especially during outbreaks of plague and other epidemic diseases; people and goods could expect to be inspected. In any case, absolute monarchs and despots needed information about the comings and goings of their enemies. The FBI, CIA, MI5, and KGB have many forerunners, although most earlier networks of surveillance were concerned with security and control rather than with health.

Once statutes are on the books, they need to be policed, and Medical Officers of Health, factory surgeons, port medical authorities, and the host of other individuals concerned with the public's health became a visible part of 19th-century Western society. The starkest instance of the police functions of public health officials, as well as ordinary medical practitioners, is seen in the development of the concept of the notifiable disease. A number of local communities had insisted that cases of smallpox had to be reported to central authorities. From the 1880s, in the wake of bacteriology, national schemes were inaugurated and several diseases were identified as contagious and public health risks. Smallpox, scarlet fever, typhoid fever, and, eventually, tuberculosis and syphilis became diseases in which the risk to the general public was deemed greater than the value of privacy and individual treatment by a medical man. Medical practitioners were required to add surveillance to their other tasks (resistance to the bureaucracy lessened after they were paid for filling out the forms), and although MoHs and equivalent officials in different countries occupied the front line, all doctors were expected to serve in the ranks.

The range of legal, medical, and ethical issues involved in surveillance is starkly seen in the famous case of Mary Mallon (1869–1939), 'Typhoid Mary'. This Irish-born woman served as a cook for a series of wealthy New York families in the first decade of the 20th century. She was completely well but displayed all the characteristics that Robert Koch had recently identified as the 'carrier state', that is, she shed the bacteria of typhoid fever without suffering from the symptoms herself. She infected members of several families, and the isolated outbreaks were investigated by public health officials. A female immigrant, with limited education, and conscious of no wrong-doing, Mary was nevertheless a public health hazard, and incarcerated for her 'crime'.

Surveying was the activity of officials intent on uncovering new associations; surveillance became the duty of all doctors who encountered a patient with a notifiable disease. Statistics became the expertise of those especially trained to understand the nature of correlations and causations. The modern public health movement emerged simultaneously with statistical societies, and for many of the same reasons. Both were responses to industrialization, and the movement and the societies were peopled by many of the same concerned individuals.

Although the mathematics of probability had been developed from the late 17th century, its contemporary mathematical partner 'statistics' was in the early 19th century much less sophisticated. Statistical societies were mostly devoted to collecting many observations and presenting these in tabular form. The introduction of civil death registration in many European countries led to annual presentation of tabular causes of death, and at the same time required international attempts to standardize diagnostic categories. Although many of the symptom-based disease categories (such as 'fever' or 'jaundice') had to be abandoned as diseases in their own right, nosology still maintained its importance, as doctors both nationally and internationally wanted to be certain of the diseases that were put on death certificates or annual hospital reports.

Of equal lasting importance, 'significance' entered statistics, originally through the work of Charles Darwin's cousin, Francis Galton (1822–1911). Galton became intrigued with the nature of heredity, and developed mathematical methods to examine the relative contributions of both parents, as well as grandparents and other ancestors, to the inherited makeup of an individual. As the father of eugenics, he was especially concerned with what he perceived as the differential birth rate between feckless poor and responsible middle-class parents. He measured many human attributes, such as height, longevity, muscle strength, and 'success' in life. He put inheritance into the public health equation, in a field that had hitherto mostly concerned itself with environmental issues such as overcrowding and dirt. After Galton, both 'nature' and 'nurture' had to be considered.

Although Galton trained in mathematics and medicine (he never practised), it was his disciple Karl Pearson (1857–1936) who placed statistics at the centre of both experimental science and clinical medicine. Our notions of significance, with its 'p' value (the level of 95% confidence that the variable being measured is correct), owe much to Pearson. He studied inheritance in tuberculosis and alcoholism, but he was mostly interested in the role of inheritance in evolutionary biology. His pupils and followers placed mathematics at the centre of epidemiology and the evaluation of new therapies through the development of the clinical trial.

These 20th-century developments have transformed the simple surveys and tabulations of earlier public health advocates. But the 19th-century message of those concerned with diseases within the community has stuck: facts are important, and so are numbers. The *méthode numérique* that Louis had used so well within the hospital had resonance outside of it. Data had to be evaluated, in the hospital, community and the laboratory, and the mathematical and statistical tools to effect this have gained increasing importance in modern health research and disease prevention.

Chapter 5
Medicine in the laboratory

Making medicine scientific

Western medicine has always fancied that it was 'scientific', but what that means has changed. The Hippocratics would have counted themselves in the ranks of science (the Greeks would have used words like 'natural philosophy'). So would the many followers of Galen. The medicine they practised had two fundamental 'scientific' attributes.

The first was an underlying rationality, which surmised that, given their world views, their actions – the diagnoses and therapies – made sense. This is of course a relativistic view of science, since astrological medicine is also rational, assuming that one accepts the influence of the planets and stars on human behaviour and earthly events. To dismiss it, one needs to discount the underlying principles, not the rationality that governed the whole process of reasoning.

The second was that medical practice has always been rooted in 'experience', from which we also derive the word 'experiment'. 'Experience' told doctors and their patients that bloodletting, for instance, helped, or that a thousand other remedies that seem ineffective, even disgusting, to us, were just what the doctor ordered. Historians can attribute these encounters to the healing power of nature, to the patient getting better despite, not because of, his or her treatment, or to the old logical fallacy we have already encountered: *post hoc, ergo propter hoc*. These retrospective judgements do not invalidate what historical participants interpreted as 'rational', 'scientific' medicine.

From the early-modern period, however, experience came increasingly to incorporate experiment, which was often situated in a laboratory. The word literally means a place where someone works, and laboratories were initially in people's homes, and were simply rooms set aside by those with sufficient leisure to enquire into the secrets of nature. The quintessential early laboratory, and the one most frequently illustrated, was that of the alchemist, as natural philosophers sought to learn how to turn base metals into gold. The alchemist's tools were the furnace, distiller, reagents, balance, and flasks of various sizes. Those interested in anatomy, physiology, and other life sciences would possess dissecting tables, surgical instruments, and other equipment to measure whatever parameter was under investigation. The Belgian physician J. B. Van Helmont (1579–1644) kept a young sapling in a pot for five years, watering it regularly with rain water. He then weighed the tree and its surrounding soil. The soil was more or less the same weight as when he had planted the sapling, whereas the tree then weighed 164 pounds, an increase Van Helmont attributed to the water. In Italy, Santorio Santorio (1561–1636) designed a chair in which he could carefully weigh himself, keeping a thorough tally of the weight of food and drink he ingested, and the weight of his excreta. The difference was what he lost in 'insensible perspiration', as he called it. William Harvey dissected snakes, toads, and other cold-blooded creatures, the better to observe the details of the heart-beat, in his quest to understand the 'motion of the heart' and circulation of the blood. Albrecht von Haller (1708–77) conducted an extensive series of experiments on living animals in his differentiation of irritability (the capacity to react to external stimuli, a property of muscles) and sensitivity (the capacity to feel, the result of nervous function). The experimental impulse in medicine has a long tradition, often involving the quantitative spirit. What could be measured could be known.

One tool among many that might be found in these early scientific workplaces was the microscope. There were problems, realized at the time, of distortion and aberration, and historians have sometimes dismissed microscopy before the 19th century as a plaything of rich dilettantes. Recent scholarship has shown how important microscopy was in serious scientific debates from its early use in the 17th century, above all by Antoni van Leeuwenhoek (1632–1723), a self-taught microscopist who worked as a draper in the Netherlands, and Robert Hooke (1635–1703), also from humble origins but a man who rivalled Isaac Newton in the breadth of his research. Hooke coined the word 'cell' in his *Micrographia* (1665). Once the microscope allowed individuals to witness the new world that it revealed, the technical problems were set aside as an inconvenience, compared to the possibilities its use opened up. In the 19th century, the microscope became the symbol of the medical scientist, occupying the identical role that the stethoscope had for the progressive clinician.

Cells: ever smaller

The basic unit of medical understanding of disease has become steadily more refined. Humoralism worked with whole bodies; Morgagni used the organs as his default mode; Bichat noticed how important tissues were for classifying and analysing pathological changes. Cells then became the key, and have remained central, even as sub-cellular units and molecules have since been identified as crucial constituents of the dynamics of disease processes.

The cell theory that finally triumphed from the 1830s can be seen as the foundation stone of both modern medical science and biology. The word 'biology' dates from 1801, whereas 'scientist' was not coined until 1833. These two words suggest that something fundamental changed during those decades. In the early 19th century, several theories proposed some kind of microscopic unit from which whole organisms were composed. Some of these units, such as 'globules', were actually artefacts of the microscopes then in use. The technical problems were largely resolved in the late 1820s. Descriptions appeared regularly of units that are recognizable as our 'cells', as well as their contents, especially the nucleus. Then, in the successive years of 1838 and 1839, two German scientists, Mathias Schleiden (1804–81) and Theodor Schwann (1810–82), proposed that cells are the building blocks of plants and animals, respectively. That they were both German is no accident, for much of modern biomedical research originated in Germany, within the German university system. Schleiden was an academic botanist, but Schwann, trained as a doctor, was the

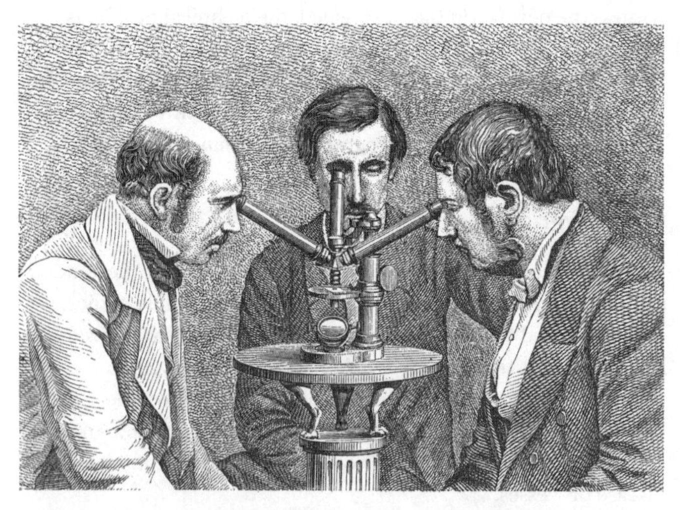

18. One of the ongoing problems with microscopy was the fact that only one person could look at the image at a time. Robert Koch made it much more public by using the camera to record images; a more companionable solution, from 1871, was this microscope, with three tubes, so providing objective verification of the magnified image

pupil of the most important teacher of medical science, Johannes Müller (1801–58). Schwann had a fabulously successful early research career, making fundamental discoveries about the nature of fermentation and digestion, as well as elaborating his cell theory. He argued that complex organisms were collections of integrated cells, and that therefore function, both normal and pathological, had to be understood in terms of the living characteristics of these entities. He believed that primitive cells, for instance, in early embryological development, or in tissues that were inflamed, could crystallize out from an amorphous fluid which he called the 'blastema'. This theory seemed to square what the microscope could reveal with his notion that life was the product of essentially a physical process.

Schwann soon abandoned his confident materialism and spent the last decades of his life in religious and philosophical speculations. His cell theory found general favour, however, and was modified and applied to medicine by others, especially by Rudolf Virchow (1821–1902), the dominant figure within 19th-century German medical science. Virchow was a life-long liberal in an increasingly militant German society, and in his youth had a touch of the political radical about him. He spearheaded a reformist group of young doctors during the revolutions that accompanied the 1848 cholera epidemic, spending a bit of time on the barricades that were thrown up by revolutionaries in Berlin. To remove him to a backwater, the Prussian authorities sent him to investigate an epidemic of typhus in Upper Silesia, now part of Poland but then within the Prussian sphere of influence. He wrote a report that the authorities did not wish to read, blaming the epidemic on social deprivation, poverty, illiteracy, and political inequality. These and similar epidemics were best controlled, he argued, through democracy, education, and economic justice. He believed that one important role of doctors was simply to campaign for such reforms. Doctors were the natural advocates of the poor, since their profession brought them into intimate contact with the economic and social causes of disease.

Virchow always maintained his interest in politics and sanitary reform, serving in the German parliament and the Berlin public health council. He liked to compare the body politic with the human body, cells becoming the body's citizens. Doctors had to confront in their daily work the adverse effects on health of poverty. This man of incredible energy also pursued his interests in anthropology and archaeology, as well as editing several journals and multi-volume books. The pathology journal he founded and edited for more than half a century is still published, known as *Virchows Archiv*. And it was primarily as a pathologist that he is remembered. Always convinced that the microscope was central to understanding disease processes ('Learn to see microscopically', he taught his students), Virchow took previous cell theories and applied them to medicine. He came to doubt that Schwann's 'blastema' was the source of new cells, such as those in early embryological development, or in inflammatory responses in the tissues, arguing instead that *all* cells come from mother cells (*Omnis cellula e cellula*). Although the slogan was not originally his, Virchow convinced the scientific world that cells do not crystallize or otherwise originate spontaneously, but that they are always the result of cell division. He elaborated his cellular pathology in the 1850s, in a series of articles, mostly in his own journals, and in 1858, then back in Berlin after seven years as professor of pathology in Würzburg, published a series of lectures, as *Cellular Pathologie*. In it he showed how cells were the fundamental units of physiological and pathological activity, and that routine clinical events, such as acute and chronic inflammation, cancer growth and spread, and bodily reactions to external stimulation such as irritation or pressure, could be fruitfully conceptualized in cellular terms. He placed the cell at the centre of pathology, even as he elaborated a more general biological principle.

Virchow made many important observations on a variety of diseases, such as phlebitis, embolism, cancers, and amyloidosis, a rare disease that is still not well understood. He also was the most influential teacher of pathology in the 19th century, and many of the subsequent leaders in the field passed through his Institute in Berlin. He carried out some active animal experiments, but much of his work was spent examining pathological tissues and cells, and relating his own findings to the clinical issues that had occurred during the patient's lifetime. He witnessed the development of new microscopical techniques, such as using microtomes to cut thin slices of tissues, the better to observe them, and stains to highlight features of cells, such as their nucleus and bodies in the cytoplasm. Although he was something of an experimentalist, experimental pathology came into its own only late in Virchow's life, with bacteriology. Virchow followed this discipline with interest but never wholeheartedly endorsed germ theory.

Germs: the new gospel

In the medical pantheon, there are few saints more revered than St Louis – Louis Pasteur (1822–95). That he was not even a qualified doctor, but trained in physics and chemistry, says much about the increasing importance of science for medicine. That he worked mostly in the laboratory, coming to the bedside only late in his life, to watch while doctors injected his rabies vaccine, reminds us of the place of the laboratory in our total picture of modern medicine.

Traditionally, the germ theory has been seen as the beginnings of effective, and therefore modern, medicine. Revisionist historians sometimes point out that the discovery that micro-organisms cause many of the most important historical diseases – typhus, tuberculosis, syphilis, cholera, malaria, smallpox, influenza, and many others – took decades of debate before some sort of consensus was reached. Further, so this revisionist account emphasizes, medicine remained therapeutically inept long after Pasteur was dead. The emergence of new diseases, such as HIV infection, Lassa fever, and legionnaires' disease, the widespread development of drug resistance among micro-organisms, and the increasing prevalence of non-infectious chronic diseases in Western societies, have put germ theory into another perspective. From the 1950s, Thomas McKeown (1912–88), a professor of social medicine at Birmingham, published a series of influential studies arguing that the decline in mortality rates in Western societies was primarily affected by improvements in nutrition and general standards of living, and that organized medicine had contributed little, at least until the very recent past.

Within these readings of 19th-century medicine, the work of Pasteur, Robert Koch (1843–1910), and the other proponents of microbiology, bacteriology, and their attendant laboratory disciplines might have been doing interesting research, but its fundamental significance for patients and life expectancies had been exaggerated. What exactly did they find out, and did it matter all that much?

Pasteur was not the first to see bacteria and other micro-organisms, nor the first to talk about the 'germs of disease'. But his researches, from the late 1850s, had a wonderful logic to them, and for few scientists is it easier to connect the entire career as a series of chance observations and opportunities for which the whole is greater than the considerable sum of its parts. He became interested in micro-organisms while studying crystallization, and showed that crystals of tartaric acid (a by-product of the tanning industry) made by ordinary chemical means were always optically neutral, whereas those he obtained after micro-organisms had been at work rotated polarized light. This convinced him that living organisms had special capacities, and led him to study the properties of yeast and other industrially important organisms used in baking, brewing, and fermentation. His iconic experiments on spontaneous generation occupied him for several years in the early 1860s, and had special resonance in the wake of Darwin's *Origin of Species* (1859). His famous swan-necked flasks, to exclude air-borne contamination after the solutions had been boiled to sterilize them, are part of our affectionate image of him.

To him, these experiments showed that spontaneous generation of micro-organisms does not occur, and he won the public debates with a colleague, who repeated his experiments and often found organisms swarming in the fluid. Analysis of Pasteur's laboratory notebooks has shown that Pasteur's experiments also sometimes 'failed' (i.e. had flasks with organisms in them), but that he quietly discarded these results. He was working with the hay bacillus (akin to the causative agent of anthrax) and the spore form of this bacterium is resistant to heat, so one would expect 'negative' results to Pasteur's experiments. By suppressing these, Pasteur got the better of his opponents. He always had the most amazing knack of backing the right horse, and sticking to his guns.

Alongside his spontaneous generation experiments, Pasteur worked actively with the role of yeasts and other micro-organisms as the cause of various fermentations: of beer, wine, or the souring of milk. Schwann and other German scientists had concluded that these important everyday reactions were merely chemical, but Pasteur insisted that they need living organisms to produce, and hence were vital processes. He provided important practical knowledge for wine-makers and brewers, as well as introducing 'pasteurization' as a means of sterilizing substances like milk, to retard their spoilage.

Such was his reputation by about 1870 that he was asked by the French government to investigate an apparently infectious disease of silkworms that was threatening the silk industry. He took his family with him, put them to work, and identified the two micro-organisms responsible, then showed how they could be prevented from doing their mischief. After this work, he increasingly began to talk about a 'germ theory' of disease, and to work on the disease-causing capacity of bacteria. Fittingly, for this non-medically qualified scientist, he tackled a disease common to animals and man, anthrax. Anthrax is unusual: unlike most bacterial infections, when animals or human beings suffer from anthrax, the bacterium can routinely be seen on slides made from the blood (the 'blood smear'). Accepting that these bacteria were the causative agents, he (and several rival workers) sought ways to 'attenuate' the bacterium, so that it might produce immunity without causing the disease. Having what he thought was a satisfactory anthrax vaccine, Pasteur did a daring thing (he was a skilled publicist, perhaps the first major scientist to court the media): he invited journalists to see the inoculation of farm animals with his vaccine, then to witness the injection of live, virulent anthrax bacillae. The public result was the death of many of the unprotected animals, but not those vaccinated (he coined this term as a general one in honour of Jenner). It was reported worldwide.

After anthrax, Pasteur lived in the public domain. He was ready for it, for his final major discovery was a treatment for rabies, a relatively rare disease, but one which killed so horribly that it provoked fear and trembling. Pasteur had to work at rabies blind, for rabies is (we now know) caused by viruses, tiny organisms which in Pasteur's time were known only through their effects. Smallpox, yellow fever, measles, influenza, and a host of other viral diseases had already made their presence known. The word 'virus' had long been used in a general sense, as a 'poison' that caused disease, but it was given its more precise biological meaning early in the 20th century, as a 'filterable virus', that is, a small agent that passed through filters that would trap bacteria and other larger biological causes of disease. Tissue culture methods and, eventually, the electron microscope made identification and classification of viruses possible.

For Pasteur, dealing with the rabies 'virus' also meant working with an agent that he did not know how to cultivate. Instead, recognizing that the symptoms of rabies pointed to some kind of infection of the nervous system, he worked with the spinal cords of rabbits, and by passing the infected material serially, learned how to make the 'poison' of rabies more or less virulent. The latent time between the bite of a rabid dog or other animal, and the development of symptoms in the victim, meant that there might be time to stimulate resistance in the person who had been bitten. There were so many imponderables that such a grant application would not get past the first hurdle of a modern funding agency, and Pasteur's whole enterprise, given what he and his contemporaries knew about rabies and viruses, would have been attempted only by a person possessed with what the Greeks called hubris. Unlike Greek tragic heroes, however, Pasteur brought off his rabies treatment, and went from scientific stardom to scientific sainthood. His first public patient, Joseph Meister, survived after being bitten by a dog which was probably rabid, and other patients were soon treated. The rabies treatment created international acclaim, with patients coming to Paris from all over Europe (time was of the essence) to receive the course of injections. It also convinced many members of the public that medical research was worthwhile, and they voted with their pocketbooks. The Pasteur Institute in Paris was funded largely by public subscription. It opened in 1888 to great fanfare and was followed by many more, throughout the French area of influence and beyond. Many of these peripheral Instituts Pasteur were devoted largely to making vaccines and other biological products: the Paris headquarters manufactured vaccines, but it also had (and has) medical research as its primary objective. Pasteur spent the last seven years of his life presiding over his eponymous institute, where he also lived, died, and is buried.

Robert Koch headed a couple of institutes as well, although his were mostly funded by the German state, symptomatic of the differences in outlook towards scientific research between Germany and the rest of the world. Relations between France and Germany were frosty after the swift defeat of France by Bismarck's Prussian forces in the Franco-Prussian War (1870–81). Science was (and is) supposed to be international and objective, cutting across barriers of race, religion, nationality, or gender. The reality has always been different, and Koch and Pasteur actually played out these national antipathies in their personal and professional

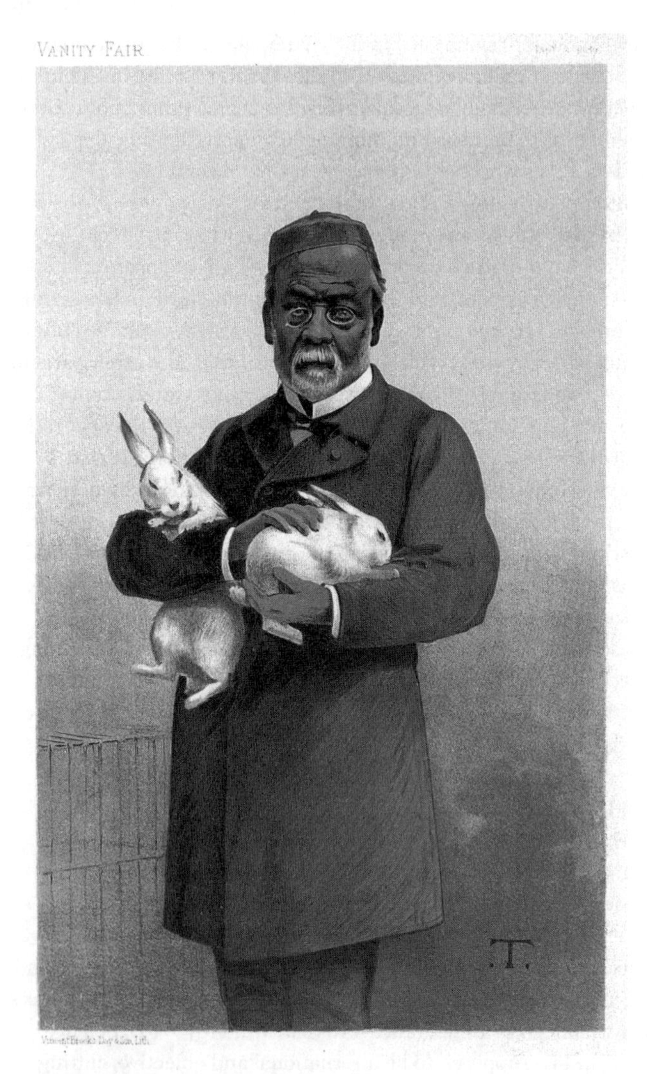

19. Louis Pasteur was one of the most illustrated scientists of the 19th century. Here, he is seen, in a *Vanity Fair* print of 1887, holding two rabbits, so important for his rabies research. Only the most famous were chosen for the series of portraits in this popular weekly magazine, published from 1868 to 1914

relationships. Pasteur sent back his honours from German states after the Franco-Prussian War, and refused to drink German beer, and Koch was eager to score as many points as he could when confronted with French microbiological and immunological findings. Their meetings at international conferences were formal but frosty.

There were ample scientific spoils to satisfy them both in the rich pickings of early bacteriology, but they possessed completely different scientific styles. Pasteur preferred to cultivate his micro-organisms in flasks, constantly changing the nutrients in the culture soup. He kept much of his research private to himself and his closest colleagues. Koch, a generation younger, was much more precise in his techniques. He introduced photomicrography, the better to present objective data to the world. He cultivated bacteria on agar-agar, a solid medium that minimized the problems of contamination. He pioneered the use of sterilization equipment, and his pupil Petri introduced the eponymous dish. Koch was a medical bacteriologist; Pasteur was a microbiologist whose fascination was with this world of the very small. Pasteur went from triumph to triumph, whereas Koch enjoyed a couple of decades of brilliant achievement and an old age in which he could not recapture the glories of his scientific youth.

Koch's first significant work involved anthrax, and as a general practitioner just after the Franco-Prussian War, he worked out this complex bacterium's life cycle, which has a spore form accounting for its ability to lie dormant in the soil for many years. The research so impressed one of his old teachers that he secured research facilities for Koch. The early results were little short of amazing: the technical innovations mentioned above, important work on the role of bacteria in the genesis of wound infections, and, crowning it all, the identification of the causative organisms of the most important disease of the 19th century, tuberculosis (1882), and of the most anxiety-provoking, cholera (1884). Both identifications were considerable technical achievements. The tubercle bacillus is fastidious, slow-growing, and difficult to stain. It was not an obvious candidate for a bacteriological cause, as a chronic disease with an extensive literature relating it to a variety of constitutional and environmental factors.

Koch reported his cholera work from India, whence he had gone after French and German expeditions had travelled to Egypt in 1883, to investigate a cholera outbreak there. The French expedition was disastrous, one of its promising young Pasteurians dying, and the expedition returning without any positive results. Koch believed that he and his group had identified the cholera organism in Egypt, but being certain of any specific organism in the gut is tricky, since there are so many bacteria always living there. Koch then went to India, the traditional home of cholera, and identified a comma-shaped organism in both water supplies and the excretions of cholera victims. Cholera had been perceived so much as a disease of filth, foul water, and high water tables that Koch's identification of a specific organism was only slowly accepted. The leading German hygienist, Max von Pettenkofer (1818–1901), had his own theory of the necessary interaction of several causative factors, of which the 'germ' was only one. In a famous gesture, he publicly swallowed a flask of Koch's bacillus, and developed only mild diarrhoea, but nothing like the full-blown disease of cholera. The pros and cons of Koch's bacillus were still being learnedly debated in the 1890s. A partially effective cholera vaccine prepared in India from the bacillus by the Russian-born bacteriologist Waldemar Haffkine (1860–1930) helped to turn the tide, and its spread by the oral-faecal route seemed to answer most of the epidemiological issues.

By the 1890s, scientifically attuned medical opinion on germ theory had shifted, and most debates were whether some specific organism caused some specific disease, or, as more was learned about immunology and the pathophysiology of infection, about the nature of bacterial toxins. The principle of the germ theory had been integrated into medical textbooks, and most medical

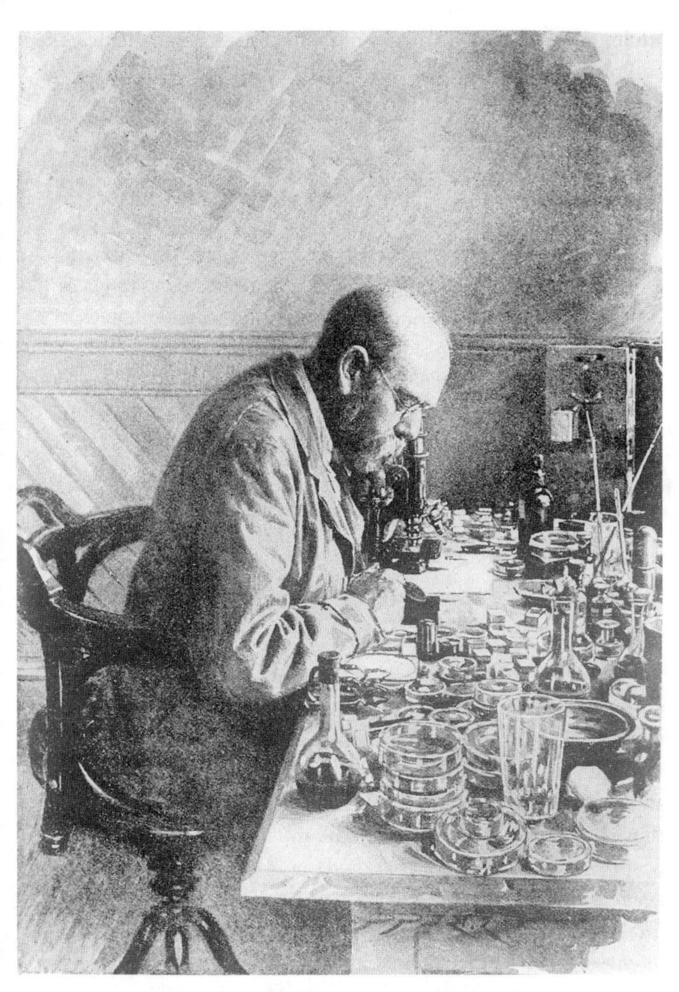

20. Robert Koch was often depicted with his microscope. Here, in South Africa in 1896–7, he is shown as a studious scientist in his laboratory, surrounded by the other tools of bacteriology, such as flasks and Petri dishes. The laboratory could be anywhere where Western science was practised

students would have learned it in their studies. Some medical men still rejected it, of course, and others thought that bacteria might be partially instrumental in infectious diseases, but hardly sufficient. The gold standard of causation was Koch's postulates, implied but never as concisely articulated by him as by his student Friedrich Löffler (1852–1915), who wrote of diphtheria:

> If diphtheria is a disease caused by a micro-organism, it is essential that three postulates are fulfilled. The fulfilment of these postulates is necessary in order to demonstrate strictly the parasitic nature of a disease:
>
> 1. The organism must be shown to be constantly present in characteristic form and arrangement in the diseased tissue.
> 2. The organism which, from its behaviour appears to be responsible for the disease, must be isolated and grown in pure culture.
> 3. The pure culture must be shown to induce the disease experimentally.

But the gold standard was hard to achieve in many diseases, and the more bacteriologists and immunologists learned about the pathophysiology of infection, the more subtle the whole process was revealed to be. Bacteria could easily be cultivated from the skin, gut, pharynx, or bodily fluids of people with no obvious signs of disease, and many of these bacteria were identical with those that in other individuals were implicated in disease. Sceptics of the whole process could point to the fact that many germs which one doctor identified as causative, other doctors doubted. Germs were associated with many conditions that were later assigned to other causes. Koch himself identified the 'carrier' state, important in the case of Typhoid Mary, in which a pathogenic germ was 'harboured' by a completely healthy individual. Outbreaks of many diseases, when investigated, threw up intricate issues of why some people succumbed to a disease, and others, similarly exposed, went scot-free. The viral diseases behaved like 'germ' ones, but their agents could not be seen.

A number of diseases that we now recognize as viral had bacteria proposed as their causative agents. Much had to be taken on trust, and doctors did disagree.

Germs, medicine, and surgery

Despite the disagreements and no little nonsense in the name of science, the trust was justified, for two theoretical and two practical reasons. Of the theoretical, neither was entirely new, but both found their full realization after germ theory. The first was the separation between the cause of disease and the patient's body. Germs were external, and although the individual's response needed to be understood through events inside the body, the cause had to be identified elsewhere. The disease was something that happened to the patient, and although the blame culture of illness hardly disappeared (and is still strong, especially for sexually transmitted and so-called lifestyle diseases), the gap between patient and cause made it easier for doctors to develop objective criteria for diagnosis.

The second theoretical implication for germs was the heightened notion of disease specificity. The earlier sanitarian movement approached most epidemic diseases as of a piece, capable of changing their character as they moved through a community. 'Filth disease' was for Edwin Chadwick a single diagnostic category, whether it manifested itself as typhus, typhoid, cholera, erysipelas, scarlet fever, or any other of the epidemic diseases that spread through the overcrowded, urban poor. Germs provided a biological basis for the distinctiveness of the different 'fevers', and finally rendered fever a sign of disease, not the disease itself. Disease classification had become a major medical issue after routine registration of death (and its causes) became common throughout industrialized nations. International interest in major epidemics, above all cholera, increased the need for these registers of causes of death to be understandable across national boundaries, and concern with nosology was merely part of the extensive effort to make scientific and medical vocabularies more precise.

The practical reverberations of germ theory were extensive, but two ought to be highlighted. The first was antiseptic, followed by aseptic, surgery. The use of the anaesthetic agents ether and chloroform from the 1840s had transformed the priorities of the surgeon, now that pain could be controlled. That these two substances were the products of chemical investigations highlights the ongoing importance of the laboratory for clinical practice. Ether anaesthesia was, incidentally, the first major American breakthrough in medicine, although its introduction was fraught with gothic tales of priority disputes, failed attempts at patents, and sordid ends to promising careers. The first public demonstration of surgery under ether took place in the Massachusetts General Hospital on 16 October 1846. News spread to Europe as fast as boats could carry it, and national medical histories are full of local 'first' operations using the new substance. Chloroform followed within a year, and the search was on for other agents that could render patients pain-free.

No medical innovation is ever without contention, and anaesthesia was no exception. Its use in childbirth was resisted by a few who believed that the Biblical injunction to Eve meant that childbirth should be painful; some military doctors thought that wounded soldiers needed the stimulus of pain the better to endure the operation; and a few deaths during anaesthetic administration alerted doctors to the dangers of the substances. These issues are sometimes emphasized in the historical literature, but the rapidity with which the new possibility of pain control spread, both among doctors and their patients, is the most striking aspect of anaesthesia's early history. Giving surgeons more time to operate made conserving tissue easier, but the longer exposure of the open wounds to the air also increased the possibility of post-operative infection. Consequently, anaesthesia enlarged the range of operations surgeons could perform, but not necessarily the chances of a patient's surviving the ordeal.

Anaesthesia provided the basis of one aspect of modern surgery. Antisepsis, and especially asepsis, provided the second. Antiseptic surgery was pioneered in the late 1860s by Joseph Lister (1827–1912). Lister was of Quaker stock. His father helped develop the achromatic microscope, so he grew up in a scientifically orientated household. He was reputedly present at the first public operation in Britain using ether, performed by the professor of surgery at University College Hospital, Robert Liston (1794–1847). Lister published substantial papers on microscopy while still a medical student, and after graduating from University College London, he headed to Edinburgh to further his surgical studies. There he married his professor's daughter and spent almost two decades in Edinburgh and Glasgow, during which time he introduced his system of antiseptic surgery, in 1867.

Lister was inspired by Pasteur's researches on the role of micro-organisms in fermentation, putrefaction, and other vital processes, and cited Pasteur in his original publication. Combining Pasteur's insights with the knowledge that carbolic acid (phenol) was successfully used to disinfect sewage, he used carbolic dressings on surgical wounds to show that compound fractures (that is, where the broken bone perforated the skin and was thus exposed to the atmosphere) could be successfully closed with this treatment. The usual alternative for a compound fracture was amputation, so poor were the surgical attempts to close it and thus save the limb. Lister's rationale was complex, and he later reconstructed his early work to make it appear that his antiseptic system was rooted in a germ theory of wound infection. It was actually based on a belief that dust particles in the air transmitted the sources of contamination (Pasteur's spontaneous generation experiments had excluded dust from his flasks), and that by dressing the wounds with carbolic-soaked dressings, he excluded the sources of wound infection.

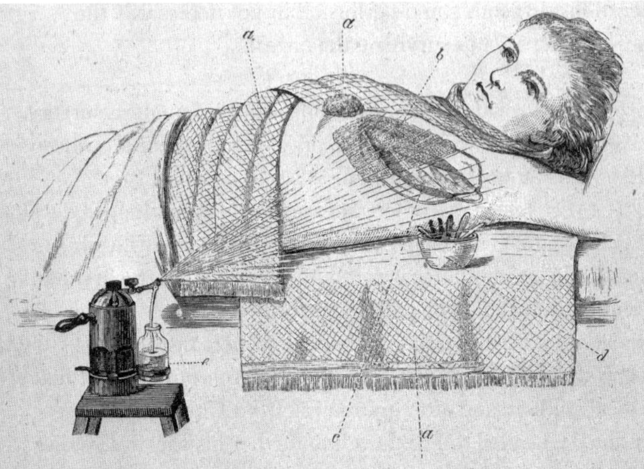

21. The preparation of a patient for a mastectomy, demonstrating how cumbersome and messy Joseph Lister's antiseptic surgery actually was in practice. The illustration is from a book (1882) by one of his disciples, Sir William Watson Cheyne

Lister's system worked and he began teaching it to his students. A number of surgeons rejected it, especially those who had already been achieving good surgical results through simple cleanliness. The Franco-Prussian War offered a good, if unplanned, comparative trial, since German surgeons had begun to take up his measures, and French ones had mostly resisted. The German surgical experience of the war was much superior to the French, and Lister's name began to be associated with a particular kind of surgical technique. Lister himself was always a fairly conservative surgeon and continued to confine himself to the traditional domains of surgery: the limbs, joints, bladder, and superficial parts of the body.

Lister continued to modify his antiseptic regime, introducing a carbolic spray and changing the routine of after-care for the surgical wound. He continued to get good results and acquired an international reputation. He and Pasteur had great respect for each other, frequently appearing on the same platform at international medical meetings that were increasingly common in the latter decades of the 19th century. As appreciation of the role of bacteria in wound infections grew, his own system gradually changed its theoretical justification and became more closely identified with the new science of bacteriology. Antiseptic surgery had a limited life, in any case. It was soon replaced with aseptic surgery, the aim not being to kill contaminating germs, but to exclude them in the first place. Asepsis excluded bacteria as completely as possible, by sterilizing equipment, instruments, dressings, the surgeon's hands, and the patient's skin. It worked on the general principle that the tissues of the body are germ-free to begin with, and if bacteria could be excluded during the operation, the wound would heal naturally, by what surgeons had long called 'first intention': healing of the wound without pus formation. Aseptic principles finally opened the three major body cavities – abdomen, thorax, and cranium – to the scapel, and surgery became the glamour speciality during the last third of the century. Techniques that Koch and others had introduced into the bacteriological laboratory found their natural application in the operating theatre, increasingly a separate, carefully regulated space in hospitals.

As surgeons operated on the previously forbidden cavities, their initial success rates were very low, as other problems, such as excessive bleeding and infection, emerged. (The gastro-intestinal tract, for instance, is open to the outside world at both ends, so the bowels are not sterile like most internal parts of the body generally are.) Knife-happy surgeons became convinced of the adage 'A chance to cut is a chance to cure', as many conditions that physicians had been able to diagnose but not to do much about seemed suddenly to be amenable to radical treatment. We should remember the early mortality of heart transplants before we

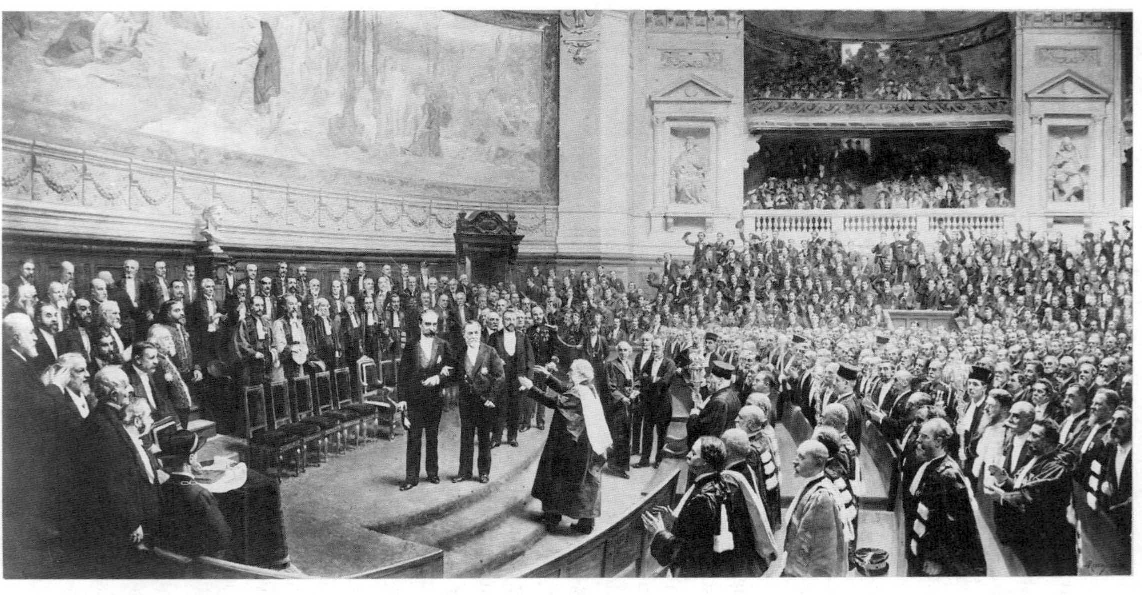

22. Medical scientist as hero: Louis Pasteur's 70th birthday in 1892 was a focus of international acclaim. Here, Joseph Lister greets the Master, before an audience of thousands

condemn a previous age, but the structures of modern-day audit were not in place, individual surgeons had relationships with individual patients, and conditions that we would not judge surgical were subjected to the knife. Thus, ovaries were removed for hysteria or menstrual pain, large segments of bowels for constipation or chronic tiredness, and tonsils were removed routinely, as a prophylaxis against all sorts of childhood complaints. The doctrine of 'focal infection' enjoyed great vogue during the early 20th century, and was used to justify the removal of portions of bowel, teeth, tonsils, and other organs for all manner of ailments, including insanity.

Modern surgery was thus built on the new power relations between surgeons and patients. Surgeons could do more and patients needed to believe in their surgeons. The historical literature tends to emphasize the outlandish operations, or those with high mortality rates and little chance of success. Looking at the impressive technical developments within surgery in the half-century before World War I, it can be seen that surgical technique grew faster than the support network (blood transfusion, antibiotics to counter infection, intensive care room monitoring), and that the ethical standards that (mostly) govern modern medical and surgical practice were not in place. There was wide variation in diagnostic fashions as well as technical ability among surgeons, so it behoved patients to choose their surgeons well. It still does.

The second major practical legacy of bacteriology was the ability to understand the sources and patterns of infections and epidemic diseases, and to react appropriately: laboratory medicine informing community medicine. Bacteriologists were 'experts' in ways that old-style sanitarians were not, and therefore they had more clout with governments and politicians. Chadwick advocated 'clean' water, but what constituted clean changed with the realization that specific pathogenic bacteria were transmitted by water, and therefore water needed to be analysed before passing it fit to be drunk. The same goes for food additives, meat quality, air purity, and the host of other things that we consume. Scientists have taken the lead in defining these things, and have provided a basis for an all-encompassing public health.

Physiology: the new rigour

Bacteriology was the medical science with the most impact on the lives of ordinary individuals during the late 19th century. Experimental physiology aroused the most tangible outcry, since physiologists began systematically to operate on living animals. Bacteriologists used a lot of animals too, but their experiments did not arouse the emotion that experimental physiology did, especially in Britain, where physiology was better developed than bacteriology.

The Germans created institutes in all the medical sciences, the most notable one in physiology being that of Carl Ludwig (1816–95) at the University of Leipzig, where students from all over the world trained. Ludwig was one of a group of four young physiologists who during the revolutionary year 1848 issued a manifesto, declaring that all the problems of physiology could be solved by the systematic application of physics and chemistry. Two of the others in the group went on to head physiology institutes in Berlin and Vienna, and the fourth, Hermann von Helmholtz, eventually turned to physics. In addition to important work in electromagnetism and conservation of energy, he was an expert in the physiology of the special sense organs, and the physics of hearing. All four of the group maintained their basic physical orientation to physiology. Ludwig's principal research interests were the functions of the heart and kidneys, and his textbook was popular both in the German-speaking lands and abroad, through translations. German was the language of medical science in the period, so even the German edition had a wide international readership. The laboratories of these and other German physiologists began to acquire a modern look, as scientists availed themselves of the latest technological aids. Helmholtz invented the ophthalmoscope, and Ludwig developed the kymograph, a turning drum connected to a recording device that allowed the measurement of continuous functional variations, such as the pulse, muscle contractions, or changes in tension. The graphical recording of vital events has increasingly characterized biomedical research and clinical medicine.

Physiology flourished in Germany, although the pre-eminent physiologist of the century was French: Claude Bernard (1813–78). He went through the Paris medical school, and recognized that the clinical orientation that dominated it could only go so far in understanding disease mechanisms or in searching for new remedies. An unhappy marriage at least brought him a dowry to allow a career in medical research, although his animal experimentations further alienated him from his wife and daughter. Bernard was above all a gifted surgical craftsman within the laboratory. His early work elucidated the role of the liver in sugar metabolism, and the function of the pancreas in digestion. He made further important discoveries in the functions of the peripheral nerves, elucidated the way in which carbon monoxide poisons, and produced a kind of diabetes through a selective destruction of a portion of the brain. He was above all intrigued by the way physiological mechanisms worked together to produce a functional whole animal. His concept of the 'internal milieu' helped explain how organisms function by keeping within a narrow range many physiological parameters, such as temperature, the ionic salts in the bloodstream, and blood sugar. His concept was later renamed 'homeostasis' by the American physiologist Walter Cannon, and it remains fundamental to our understanding of health, disease, and evolution.

Bernard had a philosophical turn of mind, and he summarized his own research career, as well as developing a philosophy of medical research, in his classic *Introduction to the Study of Experimental Medicine* (1865). It remains a book well worth reading. In it,

Bernard argued that the laboratory was the true sanctuary of medical science. In the hospital, where sick patients need care, and the number of variables means that observations are only piecemeal, no real experimental science can flourish. Only in the laboratory can the experimenter keep variables constant, so that changes can be unambiguous. Pasteur once opined that chance favoured the prepared mind, and Bernard was alive to the role of chance observations leading him into fruitful investigative paths. For instance, rabbit urine is usually alkaline and turbid; observing the urine of fasting rabbits turn acidic, he reasoned that they were metabolizing their own tissues. This led him to investigate the digestion of various foodstuffs. His philosophy of discovery was what is now called the hypothetico-deductive method: a scientist forms an hypothesis about some phenomenon. He then deduces what might happen in consequence and experiments to see if his hypothesis is correct, being careful to put aside his expectations while doing the experiment. Bernard likened this to a hat being the thinking facility. The good scientist puts his hat on the rack while doing the experiment, but he does not forget to put it on again when leaving the laboratory, to think about what he has seen, and what it means. On the basis of his experiment, he can confirm, reject, or modify his hypothesis, and then, if necessary, further test it.

For Bernard, the three pillars of experimental medicine were physiology, dealing with normal function; pathology, investigating abnormal function; and therapeutics, concerned with discovering effective remedies. His own researches contributed to each of these fields, but the important point was that each had to be rigorously experimental, a goal achievable only in the laboratory. Field work, autopsies, and bedside observations could provide the raw data and help formulate pertinent questions. The essential goal of science, however, was to elucidate mechanisms and causes. Bernard and Pasteur were friends, and the former recognized the importance of Pasteur's work, even if he died before its full potential was realized. Pasteur saw in Bernard an eloquent apologist for the experimental method within medicine: the future.

Although experimental physiology took the brunt of the antivivisection movement, only in Britain was there legislation to regulate animal experimentation. The 1876 Cruelty to Animals Act initially worried medical researchers, but in fact it provided a reasonable framework within which to pursue animal-based research, and by moving research away from private laboratories within scientists' own homes, helped to institutionalize it within public and university settings. The most important tool for physiologists was anaesthesia. Not only did it prevent pain in experimental animals, it also made operative conditions easier. Antiseptic and aseptic techniques also served physiology, another instance of clinical medicine and experimental science reinforcing each other.

A number of medical specialties benefited from physiological research. Neurology, for instance, relied on work on cerebral localization. Cardiologists made use of animal research on cardiac contraction and the regulation of the heart-beat. Endocrinology (the medical specialty of the glands) was made possible by the discovery of the hormones, by two physiologists, Ernest Starling (1866–1927) and William Bayliss (1860–1924). Medical and surgical specialties were not simply 'natural'; they also relied on the activities of groups of individuals keen on careers and prestige. But medicine and surgery by the outbreak of World War I could call upon much knowledge that had been gained within the laboratory, and increasingly by individuals whose careers were within medical science, not clinical medicine.

Chapter 6
Medicine in the modern world

What happened next?

The first five chapters have been roughly chronological, from Hippocrates to the outbreak of World War I. This chapter deals with the medicine of the past century. In it, we shall look briefly at the current relevance of each of the five 'kinds' of medicine: bedside, library, hospital, community, and laboratory. Each has a place within the budgets of modern healthcare and the lives of patients and doctors.

The driving force behind modern medicine has been cost. The most urgent question of medical care of the last generation or two has too often been: Is it affordable? This question crosses national boundaries, and is applicable to tax-paid schemes such as Britain's National Health Service (NHS), private insurance and fee-based care in the United States, or basic health functions and medical aid in Africa. Health 'need', no matter how it is measured, seems infinitely elastic. The more that is available, the greater is the demand. Spiralling medical costs have shaped modern medicine. At the same time, medical effectiveness has increased in ways that even visionaries of the past would not have acknowledged. Thus, concern with efficiency has come to the fore. Medical care has become big business, and has acquired many of the strategies of international corporations. Indeed, many of the suppliers of medical care *are* international corporations, driven by profit motives. Business leaders point out that a corporation that provides shoddy or over-priced products will lose out to its competitors. Critics of Modern Medicine, Inc., point out that mending bodies and preventing disease should not be like repairing automobiles or selling toys. There is ongoing debate but few points of agreement.

Bedside medicine: the Hippocratic legacy

Hippocrates remains a much-invoked figure today. Healers of all stripes, from mainstream Western doctors to many kinds of alternative healers, claim him as their founding father. Two interconnected aspects of the Hippocratic image continue to attract: the holism of humoralism, and the importance of the patient.

Holism has once again become a mantra in recent times. Most commentators see it as a reaction to the continued reductionism in modern medical science. First bodies, then organs, then tissues, then cells, now molecules. We have institutes of molecular medicine, just as 19th-century German universities created institutes of physiology, bacteriology, or pathology. Looked at dispassionately (people are rarely dispassionate about their health or healthcare), molecular medicine simply represents the culmination of a trend that had motivated doctors since at least the 17th century to push back the level of analysis of disease. It is part and parcel of what can legitimately be described as the progress of medicine and medical science.

This constant aim at ever lower levels of analysis has not met with universal approval, even among medical practitioners. The feeling that 'we murder to dissect' has been around longer than the author of the sentence, the Romantic poet William Wordsworth (1770–1850). The Romantics waged war against the inexorable analysis of the parts at the expense of the whole, and following the horrors of World War I, and the rapid growth of specialization within medicine, many doctors felt that a new foundation was needed for medicine. The holism movement that developed adopted Hippocrates as its figure-head, and attempted to conceive disease in general terms such as the patient's constitution. Doctors encouraged their charges to return to nature, to eat simple foods, wear practical clothes (or none: nudism was also part of the movement), and live lives that were attuned to the dictates of nature. The movement attracted a number of famous doctors, especially those suspicious of experimental science and of medical specialization, and resulted in a number of concrete experiments. In Britain, the most famous was the Health Centre at Peckham, South London, opened in 1928. Its founders argued that medicine had for too long emphasized disease, and that the biology of health ought to be its primary concern. It encouraged family life, and for families to come regularly to the centre, to participate in its physical and social activities, not a million miles away from those on offer at the contemporary fitness club.

The holism movement within medicine was never more than a minority voice, and its influence quickly evaporated after World War II, partly because it had been espoused by a number of leading Nazi doctors, and partly because the new range of biologicals and miracle drugs, above all, insulin, penicillin, and cortisone, promised that experimental research might indeed cure all ills. The 'golden age' of modern medicine dominated the middle third of the 20th century, and doctors enjoyed an unprecedented era of prestige and trust. Infectious diseases were believed to be more or less conquered, psychiatric disorders were to be controlled by the new thorazine and the other brands of antipsychotic drugs, and cures for cancers were on the horizon.

It is no coincidence that general practice, or family medicine, was at a low ebb during these decades. In Britain, it was assumed that general practitioners were made up of those not good enough to become consultants in the new NHS, or private consultants in Harley Street. Medical or surgical specialization was the presumed aim of any medical student, for specialists were the elites who ruled the profession.

From the 1960s, things began to change. The Vietnam War sparked a protest generation which was suspicious of all forms of power. At the same time, the attacks on the professions, as cryptic trade unions, concerned with income and freedom to do as their members pleased, began to gather pace. The Austrian social critic Ivan Illich (1926–2002) launched his attack on educationalists, doctors, and other professionals, with doctors creating as much disease ('iatrogenesis') as they purported to cure. Illich urged people (not 'patients', or even 'clients' as they have recently become) to take control of their bodies and health. Illich was only one of a number of counterculture advocates (in Britain, Mrs Thatcher from a right-wing perspective began her own attack on the professions) who forced doctors and other professionals onto the back foot. Doctor–patient relationships began to change, with power shifting in the direction of patients.

Two developments among many can be mentioned as evidence. First, the nature of general practice began to be reformulated. It had always been more concerned with the 'whole patient' than had the specialties, and Michael Balint (1896–1970), among others, highlighted how many psychiatric disorders (such as depression, anxiety, insomnia) were being dealt with by general practitioners. Balint was instrumental in the reformulation of family medicine as a vibrant and important aspect of medical care. It became an academic discipline, and gained prestige within the medical hierarchy. The irony that general practice raised itself up by becoming a 'general' specialism, with its own training protocols, examinations, and (in Britain) a Royal College, has not been lost on commentators. The fact remains that it was adapting to the demands of the times.

The second development was the emphasis on primary care in developing countries. International medical aid from the time of the League of Nations, formed after World War I, to the World Health Organization (WHO) and related international agencies created after World War II, had emphasized vertical, technologically driven programmes. Malaria, smallpox, schistosomiasis, hookworm, onchocerciasis (river blindness), and other specific diseases had been singled out for attention. The smallpox campaign succeeded completely, and other programmes had some significant successes, but that for malaria failed, spectacularly.

At an international conference of WHO held at Alma Ata, Kazakhstan, in 1978, the emphasis officially shifted to horizontal programmes, that is, primary care, education, and basic infrastructure, instead of specific vertical programmes aimed at individual diseases. Vertical programmes have not been completely abandoned, but the shift recognized the importance of the general over the specific, in terms of sustainability and efficiency. It prioritized individual health practitioners educating, diagnosing, and treating individual patients and their families.

Hippocrates is a sufficiently secure icon that anyone can identify with him with impunity. Nevertheless, many of the values of bedside medicine in the Hippocratic corpus have re-entered the mainstream.

Library medicine: what price information?

The coming of books in the 15th century transformed medical knowledge. Two centuries later, medical and scientific journals changed the timescale. Books might be rushed into print to communicate an exciting new discovery or theory, but they might just as well be the careful product of a lifetime's reflections. Journals, with their regular production schedule, were designed to be up-to-date. The early journals were mostly the productions of the scientific societies of the 17th century. Doctors and medical topics were well represented, and from the next century special medical journals began to appear. By the 1800s, the beginnings of an exponential growth had occurred, although since it was from a low base, it represented fewer new titles each year than we have become accustomed to. Weekly journals, such as those now called *The New England Journal of Medicine* (1812) and *Lancet* (1823), both still influential voices within medicine, allowed even speedier publication and also encouraged leaders, news items, and correspondence, all important in the formation of the modern medical profession.

The deaths of the book and the printed journal have been regularly forecast during the past couple of decades, when the computer, internet, and electronic publishing have transformed the way knowledge is disseminated. Neither has happened, and both books and journals appear at an increasing rate. The economics of publishing mean that ultimate change will undoubtedly be gradual. Nevertheless, 'library medicine' now lives like the rest of us in the computer age, and it has had at least two significant impacts on medical care.

First, the relationship between patients and their doctors has been changed by the fact that individuals now have easy access to medical information. Patients curious about the implications of a diagnosis or treatment could always ask their doctors, or take themselves to a library. The internet has made this easier, and has encouraged patients to be more involved in their own medical care. This phenomenon has merely accentuated a welcome process that has been underway for a generation or more. It requires medical personnel to be more communicative and communication skills are now taught (with varying degrees of success) in medical schools. It also creates problems, since the unregulated nature of the internet means that patients may receive partial, biased, or simply wrong information. Modern concerns with patients' rights and the ease of access to information have shifted the balance of power between doctors and many of their patients. For the most part, this is a healthy situation, and requires doctors to spend more time with their patients.

Second, patient records have been fundamentally transformed by the new information revolution. There are major issues of access and confidentiality, and any national scheme, such as the one being attempted in the UK, is extremely expensive and so far unsuccessful. The hope that each patient would have his or her own medical record on a chip is good in theory: it would make life for health personnel in accident and emergency rooms much easier, and provide doctors with the information they need wherever the patient happens to be. In the short term, at least, the scheme would work mostly for those patients who are sufficiently concerned with their health to cooperate. Access to these data by insurance companies and employers is still an unresolved issue, and the utopian ideal is likely to remain fraught.

As librarians become information officers, and doctors stare at their computer screens instead of engaging with their patients, the troubled patient may be forgiven for thinking that the brave new world is not necessarily for the best.

Hospital medicine: what price care?

Hospitals have been central to medicine since the transformation in medical thinking and education that accompanied the French Revolution. They have of course evolved during the past two centuries, in their architectural forms, organization, funding, and medical and surgical functions.

Hospital architecture has become a special subject in its own right, as social, economic, and medical demands have changed. Many hospitals in the early-modern period deliberately reflected their religious origins and aspirations. They were often built, like cathedrals, in a cruciform shape, with altars and, inevitably, a chapel. In many parts of Europe, Roman Catholicism provided both the architectural inspiration and the nursing orders which provided daily care. In Protestant Europe, more secular forms developed, and many purpose-built hospitals in Enlightenment Britain bore more than a passing resemblance to the country house. The smaller specialist hospitals, dealing with such issues as childbirth, venereal disease, smallpox, diseases of children or of the lungs or eyes, were often started in an ordinary house, taken over for the purpose. Successful hospitals would move to larger premises, sometimes simply a larger house, but increasingly into a purpose-built structure. The specific demands were not very different from those of a house: a kitchen, privies or other facilities for waste disposal, rooms for beds, and, generally, quarters for a doctor. Surgery or childbirth generally took place in the patient's ordinary bed, and sometimes this would be shared with other patients.

During the 19th century, specific medical and surgical requirements began to determine some aspects of hospital design. Pavilion wards, rectangular in shape with tall windows on both sides, had been a feature of military hospitals, and the Nightingale movement within nursing made this style of ward standard for large general hospitals. The pavilion ward had two desirable qualities: the double rows of windows made ventilation easy, in an age when miasmatic theories of disease predominated (Florence Nightingale was an ardent miasmatist and sanitarian); and the shape made nurse surveillance easy. When the Johns Hopkins Hospital was being constructed from the late 1880s, it incorporated the pavilion ward.

By then, however, there were other requirements. German university hospitals had emphasized the need for a small laboratory attached to each ward, where medical staff could perform chemical and microscopical analyses of urine, blood, and other substances. In most hospitals, the acceptance of antiseptic, and then aseptic, surgery led to special operating theatres, with appropriate sterilizing equipment. Germ theory meant that advanced hospitals needed special laboratories for cultivating sputum, blood, urine, and faeces, and cell pathology meant that tissue specimens were examined for cancer and other disorders. Biopsies taken during surgery were often read by the resident pathologist, and the nature of the operation would depend on his reading. From the end of the 19th century, X-ray equipment began to appear in hospitals, requiring space and technicians to take X-ray images and someone to interpret them. Outpatient departments also became important features of hospitals from the 1870s.

Each of these, and many more, medical and surgical innovations required adaptation of existing architectural arrangements or special consideration as new hospitals continued to be built. One should not push the analogy too closely, but there are resonances between 19th-century lunatic asylums and prisons, and between 20th-century hospitals and hotels. Both prisons and Victorian asylums were frequently built outside of cities, with surrounding walls and an emphasis on security and isolation. Hotel design and management structures have influenced modern hospitals: both have to provide food and clean linen for residents staying for variable lengths of time, and need laundry facilities as well as wholesale suppliers of food for preparation. Long central corridors with rooms coming off each side were another common feature, to say nothing of getting check-in procedures correct, including, in the United States and private hospitals everywhere, sorting out payment details.

The organizational side of hospital management has increasingly adopted business models. Early in the 20th century, American hospital administrators deliberately looked to modes of industrial production to inspire their drive for greater efficiency. Through-put, cost-cutting, and offering the client decent value for money made sense to administrators concerned with running their institutions at a profit. In Europe, most hospitals were still charitable institutions, but the same values could easily permeate, since budgets were invariably tight, and the main feature of all hospitals during the past century and a half is that of spiralling costs. In the clash between medical and economic values, the latter often dominate, no matter what the ultimate source of funding.

Costs are thus a central feature of the modern hospital, and a variety of ways have been adopted to meet them. When hospitals were largely run by religious organizations or private charity (the voluntary hospital was the principal mode of funding hospitals in Britain until they were nationalized in the context of the NHS), budgets were usually the responsibility of those who funded them, but rarely used them. Modern surgery, X-rays, and other diagnostic features meant that, from the late 19th century, the rich also had occasion to enter hospital. The British voluntary hospital solution was to build paying wards for the well-to-do, the profits of which subsidized the charitable wards. In the United States, paying wards developed earlier, and private hospitals, such as the Mayo Clinic, developed in Minnesota by the Mayo clan from the 1880s, offered advanced medical and surgical care, to those who could pay or who had private insurance. The role of insurance companies in the early 20th century is still insufficiently appreciated in medical history, and although many of the early companies emphasized their philanthropic aims, the profit motive was ever present.

Whatever the system of medical care, in Western societies, third-party arrangements are the norm in hospital payments, so large are the bills. The costs of building, heating, lighting, maintaining, equipping, and staffing these complex institutions have been an increasing concern for the past century. The guaranteeing body has been variously the state, the municipality, a religious organization, an insurance company, a charitable group, individual governors, a rich benefactor, or a combination of these. For-profit hospitals, such as those in the United States, attract much criticism, for the draconian admission policies, in which the insurance policy is more important than the diagnosis or medical need. But the drive for efficiency, and the adoption of business models, characterizes almost all modern hospitals. In the 19th century, fear of the income loss that chronic illness brought was the primary worry of working people. A debilitating illness requiring lengthy hospitalization and not adequately covered by insurance is now the fear of people who are comfortable as long as they have health.

New technologies as well as financial constraints have reduced the average length of hospital stays. Getting people out of bed quickly, even after major surgery, is now a surgical goal. There is sound medical evidence that this is a good idea, as it reduces thrombosis, bed sores, and muscle wasting, but the strategy also has economic rationale, since it reduces hospital stays. Diagnostic procedures that in an earlier age would have meant a stay in hospital are now conducted in the outpatients department.

Despite the problems, hospitals are here to stay. They have three particular features that make them indispensable: sophisticated diagnosis, acute care, and surgery. Diagnosis was the one thing that hospitals in early 19th-century France were best at, and, for different reasons, going into hospital for a battery of tests is still a common modern experience. Technology and science come together in such procedures as cardiac catheterization, to evaluate heart function; liver or kidney biopsy, to procure a piece of tissue for microscopic examination; the use of ultrasound to monitor foetal development during gestation; or the CAT scan, the computerized axial tomography, or MRI, the magnetic resonance imaging machine, two non-invasive means of visualizing structures within the body. The CAT scan and MRI use different technological and scientific principles, the former builds up a picture of the interior of the body through serial images that are combined with the use of the computer; the latter uses a strong magnetic field that is manipulated by a radiofrequency wave.

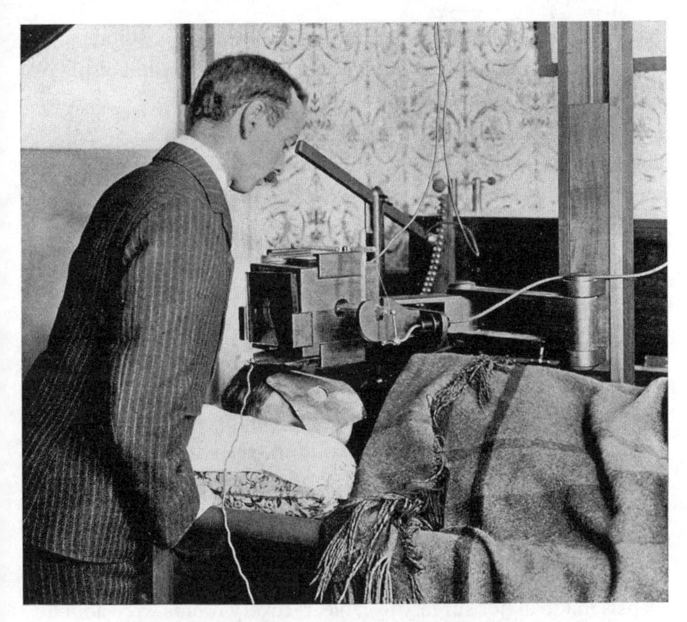

23. X-rays quickly found their uses in both diagnosis and therapy. In this image of X-ray therapy, from 1902, the apparatus has a shield around it, an unusual precaution at that time. The doctor himself is unprotected, without even a white coat as a badge of office

The two techniques have many similarities. Each innovation has been rewarded with a Nobel Prize for its developers; each produces a three-dimensional image which also shows soft tissues much more distinctly than traditional X-rays; each has dramatically furthered diagnoses and therapy, allowing, for example, needle biopsies that would previously have required invasive surgery; and each machine has been extremely expensive to build, maintain, and use. Since the MRI has fewer patient risks, and produces a clearer image of subtle soft tissue structures, it has largely replaced the CAT scan, but each in turn from the 1980s symbolized the power and costs of modern technology-driven medicine. Along with lasers, fibre-optics, and a host of other modern innovations, they have changed the face of hospital medicine, increasing what doctors can know and do, but also adding substantially to the costs of medical care.

The second feature of hospital medicine that will remain is acute care. Trauma, for instance, is not simply an important branch of military medicine, but also one that must deal with traffic accidents, knife and gun wounds, burns, and the myriad risks that modern society throws up. Terrorism has added to the visibility of the specialty. At the beginning of World War II, European countries made routine preparation for how to deal with a large number of civilian casualties; similar plans are now in place for large-scale disasters, but individual victims of accidents and acute illnesses were always part of the responsibility of hospitals.

Special places within hospitals were gradually developed to care for those acutely ill or injured. After Listerian antisepsis and asepsis made major surgery feasible, recovery rooms were added to operating theatres, and nurses who specialized in caring for surgical patients were added to hospital personnel. In the 20th century, blood pressure and other vital signs could be monitored, and with the development of intravenous fluids, and during the interwar years blood transfusion, surgical shock and other post-operative complications were dealt with more effectively. In the 1950s, continuous monitoring of the heart-beat was added to the technological equipment present there, and as heart attacks became commonly recognized as a medical emergency, coronary care units evolved to care for the acute stage. Such units are far from peaceful places for patients (or staff), and during the 1970s, it was seriously debated whether heart attack victims were better off at home, simply resting. Better control of irregularities of the heart-beat, a major cause of death in the acute phase of myocardial infarctions, as well as modern resuscitation techniques, has guaranteed the permanence of coronary care units, despite their costs and inhuman environment. Patients who have experienced strokes, diabetic coma, or other debilitating episodes are also treated in such intensive care units.

Modern surgery is also inextricably sited within the hospital. Minimally invasive techniques mean that radiologists, cardiologists, gastroenterologists, and other non-surgical specialists often perform manual procedures, but the surgeon still occupies a privileged place in the modern medical hierarchy. If Nobel Prizes are any measure of medical worth, surgeons have been under-represented, especially in more recent times. Early on, Theodor Kocher (1841–1917) won one for his work on the surgery of the thyroid, and Alexis Carrel (1873–1944), who pioneered vascular suturing, got one, although it was mostly for his research with tissue cultures. Charles Huggins (1901–97), a Canadian-born urologist, shared a Nobel Prize (1966) for showing that tumours of the prostate can be dependent on hormones. His work had been done a quarter of a century previously. The Portuguese neurologist Antonio Egas Moniz (1874–1955) shared the 1949 Prize for his work on pre-frontal lobotomy, now something of an embarrassment. In terms of helping humanity, John Charnley (1911–82), the British orthopaedic surgeon, deserved but did not receive one for his pioneering research on the technology and surgical approaches to hip replacement. Cardiac catheterization also collected one (1956), but none of the recipients was a dedicated career surgeon, reinforcing the point that surgical procedures are now performed by a variety of non-surgical specialists.

The only modern surgical Prize went to three pioneers of transplant surgery, one of the most dramatic aspects of present-day surgery, but one that has involved much basic immunological research, to control the tendency of the body to reject tissues and organs perceived as 'foreign'. Kidneys, hearts, and livers are now routinely transplanted from donors (generally dead, although a person with two healthy kidneys can spare one). Transplant surgery can accurately be described as a miracle of science and surgery, but it is also iconic for the dilemmas of modern healthcare. Receiving a foreign organ generally puts the recipient in a life-long medical relationship with his or her carers, since powerful immunosuppressant drugs must be taken on a long-term basis and they have unfortunate side effects, including increasing the donor's susceptibility to infections. More ominously, the shortage of organs for transplantation has led to an international black market, primarily through desperately poor individuals from developing countries selling their organs for use in the richer countries.

Hospitals save lives. They are also still at the centre of medical education and clinical research, but they suffer from serious structural problems. Funding is almost always an issue, and although they frequently retain the rhetoric of charity and service, they must be run like the complex institutions that they are. Antibiotic resistance among many pathogenic micro-organisms is common today, but the antibiotic-rich environment of hospitals makes them ideal places for this evolutionary phenomenon to occur. Resistance to antibiotics happens when a random genetic change in a micro-organism produces some characteristic that enables it to resist the antibiotic. In ways that Darwin would have understood, the new hereditary characteristic gives the micro-organism an advantage, and it thrives. The staphylococcus, a common bacterium which causes boils but also more serious infections, was initially susceptible to penicillin, the wonder drug of the 1940s. It soon became resistant, and as other antibiotics were developed, it acquired resistance to many of those too. We now know it by its acronym, MRSA (Meticillin Resistant *Staphylococcus Aureus*). It is a serious problem in hospitals and, since there is always movement between the hospital and the wider world, in the community as well. The causative agents of malaria, tuberculosis, and HIV have all developed resistance to many of their conventional treatments, complicating these major world diseases.

The hospital has not 'caused' this phenomenon; human agency has. But drug-resistant pathogens are now so common that modern hospitals sometimes lose their desired epithet, as 'houses of healing', and revert to that old one, 'gateways to death'.

Medicine in the community: our health in our hands

The 19th-century advocates of public health created an infrastructure throughout the Western world, developed at different speeds and sensitive to differing national ideologies. As we have seen, the movement achieved more effectiveness after the causation of infectious diseases was better understood, but the infrastructure itself was just as important. The band of individuals (MoHs; water and food analysts; sanitary, factory, and building inspectors; visiting nurses), and the ever-growing set of regulations they were empowered to enforce, were necessary to achieve the reforms that governments increasingly identified as their responsibilities. Public health was supposed to live up to its name, and extend its benefits to all members of society.

On the whole, it did, but vulnerable groups – the poor, children, the aged, and women of child-bearing age – were often targeted and stood to benefit most. While this may put an unnecessarily benevolent gloss on a good deal of late 19th- and early 20th-century public health activity, one historian has argued that war is good for babies and other young children. The war in question was the Boer War, with its disquiet that so many recruits from the slums of Britain had to be rejected from army service on health grounds, and the unsatisfactory outcome of the conflict led to fears that the British could not sustain their Empire without improving the health and fitness of their people. Similar fears fuelled the public health and pronatalist movements in other Western countries, even if the spectre of racial

X-RAY
NOW
X-RAY NOW
EASY
CONFIDENTIAL
NO
UNDRESSING
14YRS.
NOW

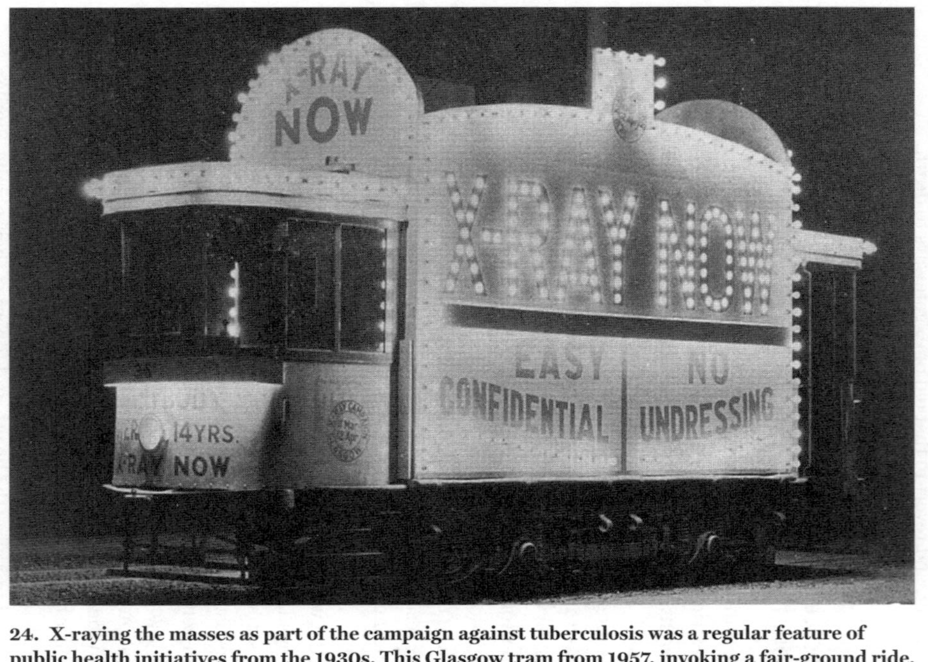

24. X-raying the masses as part of the campaign against tuberculosis was a regular feature of public health initiatives from the 1930s. This Glasgow tram from 1957, invoking a fair-ground ride, tries to make having an X-ray trendy as well as modest (no undressing, but fast and confidential)

degeneration (and a perceived birth-rate larger in the proletariat than in the solid middle classes) also stimulated the eugenics movement. Public health had traditionally been environmentalist in its orientation: get rid of dirt, overcrowding, and the slovenly morals that they engendered, and the populace would be

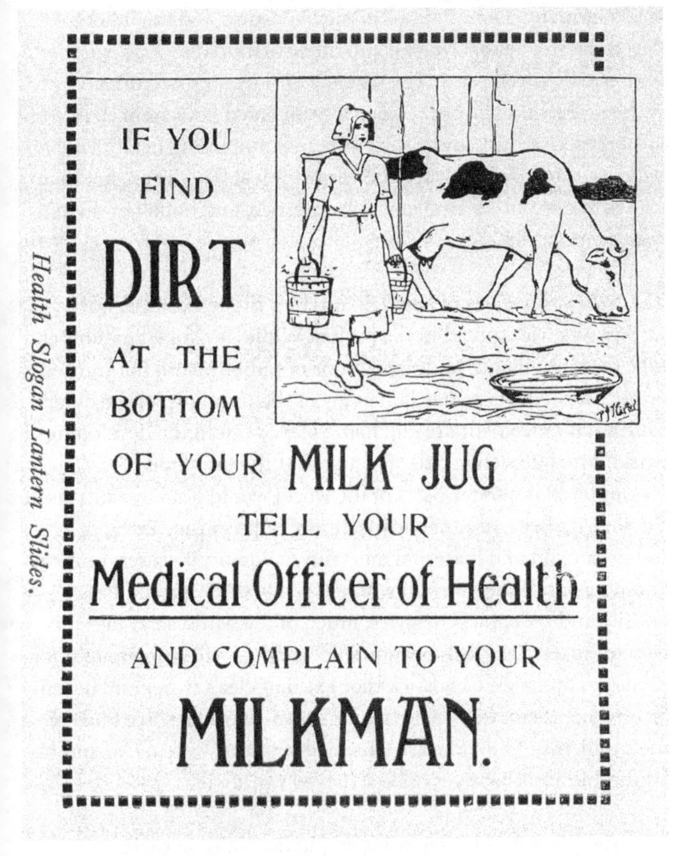

Health Slogan Lantern Slides.

25. Contaminated milk was a common source of tuberculosis spread before pasteurization became mandatory. Other potential hazards are noticed here in this 1929 lantern slide, encouraging the public to get involved by reporting to the MoH and complaining to the milkman

healthier. This older mantra was diluted by the emphasis on bad heredity, and the newer scenario that only by stopping undesirables from breeding could Western nations continue their world dominance.

As is well known, the eugenics movement reached its apogee in Nazi Germany. Their notions of racial destiny, and the inherent degeneracy of Jews, Gypsies, and other marginal groups, were barbaric in the extreme. The whole Nazi ideology was driven by a ruthless dogmatism, but it ironically included notions of the importance of fresh air and exercise in maintaining health, and a belief that tobacco and alcohol were inimical to it. There are many routes to current ideas of a healthy lifestyle, and not all of them worth emulating.

The Nazis took ideas of racial hierarchies to the extreme, but racism was widespread in the period. While developed nations can take the surveillance and regulations of public health for granted, or be incensed when they fail, many of the trappings of the older sanitarian movement are still being played out in the developing world. Much has changed, of course, but the problems encountered in poorer parts of the world would not have surprised Edwin Chadwick or other advocates in 19th-century Europe. Issues of child and maternal mortality, epidemic diseases, poverty, and poor sanitation are still with us. While the West combats obesity and sedentary lifestyles, much of the world scrabbles for enough to eat. Old-fashioned public health is still being fought for in many countries. Chadwick thought that clean water and decent arrangements for disposing of human waste would solve most of the problems of filth disease. His medical ideas were naïve, but his admirable aims have yet to be achieved worldwide.

Imperial powers did some work on public health in their possessions overseas. The British in India, for example, took cholera and malaria very seriously indeed. Neither was a uniquely 'tropical' disease, since both were known in Europe. But the discovery by Ronald Ross (1857–1932), working in the Indian Medical Service, of the role of the *Anopheles* mosquito in the transmission of malaria catalysed the development of tropical medicine as a medical specialty. Malaria occurred in temperate climates as well as tropical ones, but in many ways it fitted the model that Ross's mentor, Patrick Manson (1844–1922), elaborated as the distinct features of the diseases that the specialty had to deal with. It was transmitted by an insect, so had a more complicated life cycle and mode of spread than the bacterial diseases of the Old World. Furthermore, its causative organism was a plasmodium, not a bacterium, filling Manson's belief that worms, parasites, and other kinds of organisms were the main enemies in the tropics. Manson used Ross's work, announced in 1897 and 1898, to convince the British government to found a School of Tropical Medicine in London, in 1898. Another one in Liverpool was established a few months earlier, and a spate of institutes and schools of tropical medicine were in existence throughout the world before the outbreak of World War I.

The aim of these schools was to train medical officers to deal with the range of diseases that would confront them in Asia, Africa, and other tropical areas of the world. Tropical medicine was to make these areas safe for Europeans, to carry out their effort to Christianize, civilize, and commercialize the peoples under their dominion. Some historians have dismissed the effort as completely self-serving, carried out by governments and individuals who had no feelings for the 'natives', and who in any case merely wanted to create safe enclaves for European soldiers, merchants, planters, and civil servants. If one examines dispassionately the motives and careers of many of the key individuals involved in the effort, a much more subtle scenario is reached. At the very least, enlightened self-interest dictated that diseases needed to be controlled among all groups. In Asia, in particular, Europeans often appreciated the richness of the cultures they were controlling and exploiting. In sub-Saharan Africa, a different set of conditions obtained, accentuated by the harshness of the disease profile in

Western Africa, in particular, and the absence of a written culture. But it is historically distorting to write off medical and public health efforts in Imperial dominions as simply exploitative.

Most 'tropical medicine' before World War I was initiated by colonial powers, to serve their own possessions. The exception was missionary medicine, nurses and doctors who were concerned with spreading the message of Western health values as well as religion. Missionaries were responsible for setting up and manning health centres and hospitals in many parts of the world, and while they tended to follow established Imperial geography, there was some missionary activity outside of home-country spheres of domination. An embryonic international health movement started with the formation of the League of Nations after World War I, although much of its health-related activity was concerned with Eastern Europe and other parts of the war-torn continent. Although the United States government was reluctant to support the League, the Rockefeller Foundation and its international agencies were particularly active during the interwar years. Rockefeller officials were keen to establish Western-style institutions (medical schools, research institutions, and teaching hospitals) in areas where there was the possibility of continued indigenous support and, therefore, continuity. Europe, Mexico, and Latin America were the Foundation's primary areas of international activity, although its interest in malaria, schistosomiasis, and hookworm took Rockefeller officials to other parts of the world too.

Following the end of World War II, internationalism was finally established through the United Nations and sister organizations, especially WHO. WHO has always had admirable goals, but has struggled with the complexity of the problems it sought to confront. The dominant mode of attacking disease in the interwar years was vertical: single diseases with specific modes of transmission were singled out as the most efficient way of improving health in poor countries. Smallpox and malaria were the subjects of two major WHO campaigns in the 1950s and beyond. The malaria programme, approved at the 1955 General Assembly of WHO, was largely inspired by the availability of DDT, the insecticide that was developed during World War II and used with great effectiveness against malaria and typhus (a louse-borne disease) in the war zones.

Ever since Ross and G. B. Grassi (1854–1925) in Italy had discovered the role of the *Anopheles* mosquito in the transmission of malaria, and elucidated the life cycle of the plasmodium responsible for the disease, its control seemed straightforward. Eliminate the mosquito, through interrupting its breeding sites by draining, oiling, and employing 'mosquito brigades' to patrol the offending sites, and the disease ought to disappear. Besides, quinine could cure the disease and had long been shown to protect if taken regularly. Ross spent the last three decades of his life arguing that malaria could be prevented, if sufficient resources were devoted to it. The knowledge was there, only a lack of will (and money) prevented this desirable goal from being achieved.

For Ross, apply the vertical programme, eradicate or marginalize the disease, and a healthier workforce would achieve economic development impossible as long as the disease raged. For other malariologists, only a horizontal programme would work. The decline of malaria in Europe suggested that if a reasonable standard of living, economic development, and education were in place, malaria would fade out as a consequence. These malariologists argued that in highly malarious areas (much of Africa, for instance), the constant exposure from birth produced a population that was more or less immune. Remove this 'natural' exposure, and highly epidemic forms of the disease would thrive.

DDT seemed to consign these arguments to history. It was cheap, had a residual effect after spraying, and promised a technological fix to a complicated and widespread medical problem. Parts of worst-affected Africa were excluded from the mandate, but the

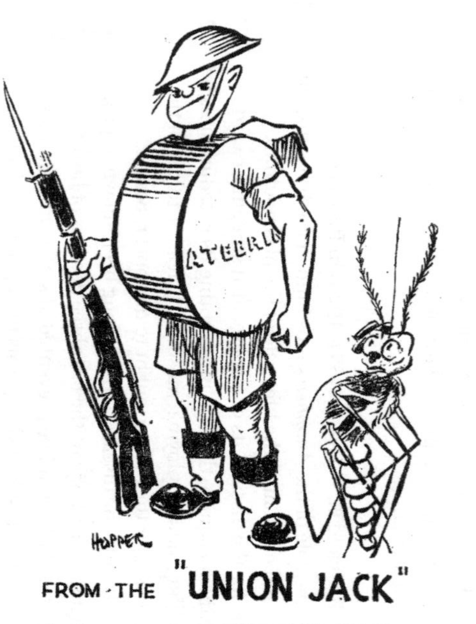

THIS MESSAGE ON MALARIA PREVENTION IS SENT OUT TO EVERY SOLDIER OF THE ALLIED ARMIES WITH THE DIRECT APPROVAL AND BY THE EXPRESS ORDERS OF GENERAL EISENHOWER, COMMANDER - IN - CHIEF OF THE ALLIED FORCES IN NORTH AFRICA. THE MESSAGE RUNS AS FOLLOWS:

«From April 22 onwards every soldier in North Africa will be given the anti-malaria tablets as already prescribed in routine orders. This regulation applies to every officer, N.C.O., and man in the Allied Forces. It must be understood that from this date onwards our troops must be equipped to fight malaria as well as the common enemy.

Every soldier should be aware that in becoming a malaria casualty, through neglect of this precaution, he is wilfully endangering his healthy neighbour because of his own infection.

Though the disease itself is readilycurable, any man who fails to take the necessary steps to avoid infection is clearly « letting down » his friends, and is thereby aiding the enemy.

Failure to take reasonable precautions is «not playing the game.» Remember that our foes, so long as they remain to contest this well-watered strip of territory, are also subject to the same malaria handicap. It is our aim to fling them out and chase them overseas. The side which combats the disease most effectively has the best chance of winning the campaign.»

Lt.-Col. J. W. SCHARFF, R.A.M.C.
MALARIAL ADVISER, A.F.H.Q.

26. Preventative medicine played an important part in the campaigns of World War II. Here, soldiers are encouraged to take their regular doses of atebrin, the most commonly used antimalarial drug of the period. Malaria was still an important disease in the Middle East, southern Europe, and the Asian theatres of war

plan was that the rest of the world would be malaria-free in a couple of decades. The campaign was approved in a fit of post-war optimism, but it was bedevilled by problems from the start. Spraying equipment would be delivered and there would be no DDT, or vice versa. Training field-workers was slow and laborious. The results in different parts of the world were variable. A growing environmental movement, spearheaded by the publication of Rachel Carson's *Silent Spring* (1962), objected to the more general effects that DDT had, and the 1960s protest movement disliked the large-scale organization of the campaign and, especially, the profits that (mostly) American firms were making from it. Finally, DDT-resistant mosquitoes began to emerge.

The malaria eradication programme was quietly converted to a focus on control in 1969, with much less fanfare than its launch. Its mistakes have since been easy targets for critical analysis, but it had achieved some successes, for instance in the Mediterranean countries of Europe, where malaria had resurged during the disruptions of World War II. Italy, Spain, Portugal, and, notably, Greece, far less developed economically than the others, were declared malaria-free during the years of the campaign. Sri Lanka came close, and the incidence of the disease in India decreased dramatically.

By contrast, the WHO smallpox eradication initiative is still heralded as a triumph of modern medicine. A triumph it was, since the last naturally occurring case of smallpox was reported in 1977, and the disease was ratified as extinct in human populations in May 1980. It was in the end the product of international cooperation and good will, not of medical science. It relied on the old (folk) discovery of vaccination, and the time-honoured methods of case tracking, isolation, and mass vaccination of populations at risk. There was no treatment save supportive measures. Smallpox could be eradicated since it had no natural animal reservoir, it was passed person to person, and could be controlled through isolation and vaccination. It was an administrative campaign, although that in no way diminishes its importance.

Vertical, single-disease campaigns are still attractive, and several have been successful. Polio is almost eradicated, and guinea worm and onchocerciasis have been counted as effective. Despite the glamour (even if the work may be routine) of single-disease strategies, the importance of primary care has also been recognized. The WHO Alma Ata conference officially mandated horizontal programmes as a necessary goal of international healthcare. In essence, this merely ratified the truism that a medical and social infrastructure is a precondition for sustainable delivery of modern public health and healthcare. Its realization has been slow, as the economic difference between the rich and the poor has increased in the past few decades, and HIV, drug-resistant malaria and tuberculosis, and wars have intervened. There have been some gains, but more setbacks, during the closing decades of the last century, and the outlook is challenging to say the least.

Some of these problems in poorer countries are simply reflections of issues in the West, where alcoholism, drug-use, resistant tuberculosis and HIV, and obesity have become major health matters. One social habit, exported from the West, threatens to be a time bomb in the coming decades: cigarette smoking. The discovery of the direct link between cigarettes and lung cancer is one of the great achievements of modern epidemiological surveillance. Lung cancer was a rare condition in earlier centuries, and its gradual increase during the interwar years was noted by many clinicians and a few statisticians. By the late 1940s, it was recognized as a serious disease of modernity, and the Medical Research Council (MRC) in Britain commissioned two individuals, a mathematically inclined clinician and a statistician, to investigate its spread, and try to determine its cause. The clinician was Richard Doll (1912–2005); the statistician, Austin Bradford Hill (1897–1991). Their own working hunches suggested that lung cancer was probably a disease of modern pollution, car exhaust fumes, or tar from road surfaces.

They began work by devising a questionnaire for patients in London hospitals diagnosed with cancer of the lung, liver, or bowel. The initial striking result was that heavy smoking was present in those with lung cancer, but not in those with the other forms of cancer. At the same time, an American study (1950), based on autopsies of patients dying of lung cancer, also found a high prevalence of smoking in the victims. Based on these suggestive findings, Doll and Hill devised a prospective study, following the health fortunes of more than 34,000 British doctors who agreed to take part in it. Because doctors must give their address changes each year to the Medical Register, an annual list of qualified medical practitioners, Doll and Hill were able to follow their cohort over the years, relating the individual's chances of acquiring lung cancer to his or her smoking habits. Since many doctors (including Doll himself) gave up the habit once the risks were exposed, the study also offered the opportunity to compute statistically the years gained by giving up the sot-weed. The final part of the study was published in 2004, 50 years later, and was written by Doll himself, with a colleague. It is probably the most remarkable 'social' experiment ever devised within medicine. It was simple in design but dogged in execution, and the results unfolded in a series of papers over half a century. By the time the 'experiment' ended, much other evidence had been produced on the health consequences of cigarette smoking, but Doll and Hill can be said to have initiated the modern movement of 'lifestyle medicine'.

The phrase is barely two decades old, but it seems here to stay. Community medicine involves surveillance, and putting the observations together has come up with a picture in which the ordinary individual has a major input on his or her health. Our choices influence our well-being. In the golden age of medicine, from the 1940s to the early 1970s, there was every confidence that,

Weight
And Alcohol
ABSOLUTELY
FIRING it DOWN
GUZZLE
GUZZLE
DIET COLA
• Alcohol is loaded with calories.
Cutting down the amount you drink can help you lose weight.
• Replacing food with alcohol can lead to health problems.
alcosense

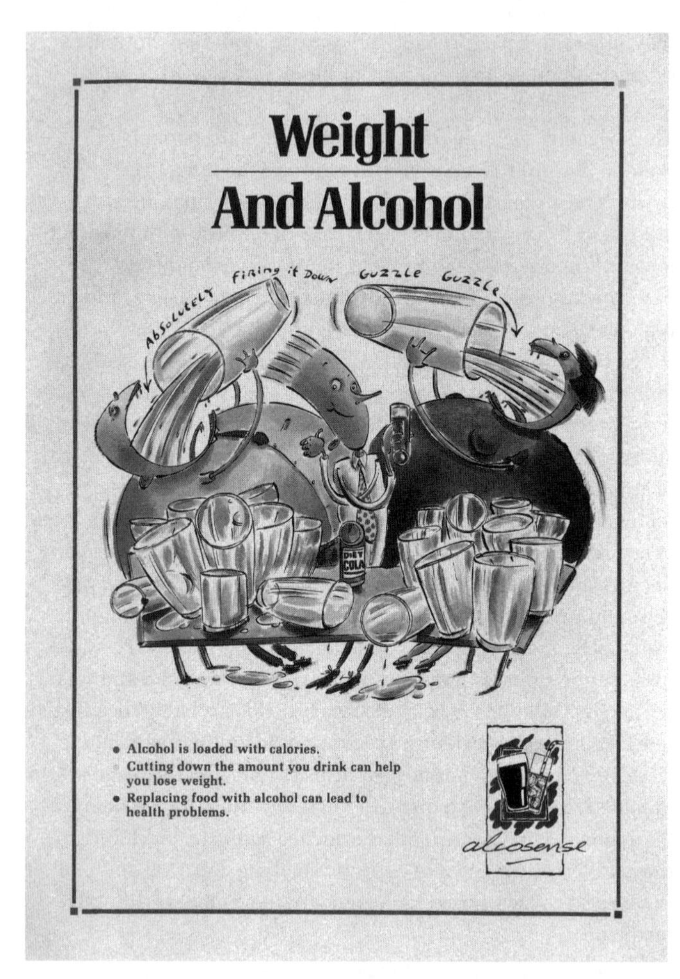

27. Lifestyle medicine from 1992, in a poster aimed both at countering obesity and the deleterious effects of excessive alcohol consumption

whatever we did, doctors could take care of us. Between surgery, antibiotics, tranquillizers, hormones, contraceptives (medicine influencing lifestyle rather than lifestyle medicine), and the range of other drugs and therapies, the promise of an age of health seemed just around the corner. Although medicine is now even more powerful, we are less confident about it. Alcoholism, smoking, drug abuse, venereal disease, obesity, fatty, high-salt takeaways, factory farming, and other dimensions of modern Western living have taken their toll. Many of these indiscretions are old, although some are new. The doctor–patient relationship has changed, and the coming of patient power has brought with it recognition of patient responsibility.

The Hippocratic emphasis on moderation reminds us that doctors have long been moral policemen. What counts as moral, and what immoral, has a tendency to change in different cultural settings. In the early-modern period, a syphilitic lesion could be a kind of badge of honour among some social groups; in the interwar period, good eating meant lots of red meat, cream, and eggs; cigarette smoking was an emblem of female emancipation. Societies change, and so does medical advice. There are good reasons to think that advice now is better than it sometimes was in the past, and even those who distrust doctors and medical science still enjoy the benefits of the surveillance and epidemiological studies that try to tease out the harmful from the beneficial. When in doubt, remember the Hippocratic injunction that health is most likely to be found in the middle way.

Laboratory medicine: still the promise of the new

The modern biomedical laboratory has never been so remote, and yet so close, to the aware, average citizen. Scientists frequently call news conferences when they think they have something important to report; all news agencies carry medical science items on a regular basis. The internet makes sophisticated knowledge available to anyone who wants to take the trouble. Despite our modern information-driven culture, surveys reveal that profound ignorance about health and science is widespread and worrisome. It has probably always been this way, and the physicist and novelist C. P. Snow's critique of the 'two cultures' had resonance before he articulated it in 1959, and still does. Snow argued that most non-scientists are less informed about the main ideas of science than scientists are about those of general culture. Ignorance is everywhere, but ignorance of science and medicine particularly so.

If the details elude them, most people know that the medicine that is practised in the 21st century has been heavily influenced by medical science. Above all, modern drug discoveries, and, more recently, the controversies surrounding the Human Genome Project and stem cell research, have been newsworthy. The latter two are beyond the scope of this historical account, but contemporary medicine has been transformed by the therapeutic power of drugs. Serendipity has played a part in the discovery of a number of them, but the laboratory has been the primary site where their therapeutic potential has been first observed. Claude Bernard's comment of the 19th century is still true: the laboratory is the sanctuary of experimental medicine.

From the late 19th century, a number of effective pharmaceutical agents began to filter through, which have had staying power. These include aspirin, phenacetin, choral hydrate, and the barbiturates. They all share the characteristic of being relatively simple chemically, amenable to the analytic methods then available. Aspirin is often mentioned as a drug that would not pass modern safety standards, given that it is a gastric irritant and can be used for suicide. Ironically, in low doses, it has been shown to be effective in preventing blood clotting, and so is used to prevent heart attacks and strokes, uses remote from what it was originally introduced for. The effect is small in the individual but significant in a large population. Its mechanism of action has been worked out only within the last generation, decades after its use was routine, as an anti-inflammatory drug and to relieve pain and fever.

Between this group of drugs and the 1920s came several chemicals and a number of biologicals, especially vaccines and antisera. None of them could compare with insulin, discovered in 1921 by a young physician turned physiologist and a medical student at the University of Toronto. Frederick Banting (1891–1941), the physiologist, obtained the use of the laboratory during the summer holidays, while the professor was on holiday. Charles Best (1899–1978), the medical student who subsequently became a distinguished physiologist himself, helped in the careful isolation of the active hormone secreted by the pancreas. Amazingly, the substance reduced the blood sugar levels of diabetics, and Banting and the absent professor, J. J. R. Macleod (1876–1935), shared the Nobel Prize almost immediately. Banting and Macleod appropriately shared their Prize moneys with Best and the chemist, J. B. Collip (1892–1965), who had helped with the purification of the substance. This was a classic one-off experiment, widespread in its therapeutic implications and fully deserving of the Prize that was quickly awarded. Within a year, commercial insulin was available, and for diabetics the new drug could be life-saving. Insulin is paradigmatic of both experimental medicine and modern medical care. Insulin controlled diabetes, it did not 'cure' it, and its victims were still left with a permanent affliction that needed daily management. Despite better ways of administering the drug and different preparations, insulin-dependent diabetes is a life-long problem with many complications which also need to be managed as they occur. Time and again, modern hopes of cure have really been the sentence of chronic care, better than the alternative, but less than early expectation. The brutal truth is that the human body is a wonderfully evolved machine, and medicine rarely does as well as nature.

Despite the ongoing issues relating to diabetes control, insulin was a major innovation, and seen as such by patients. It encouraged the general public to expect more from laboratory investigations, an attitude reinforced by success in treating pernicious anaemia. The results were not so dramatic as those of patients in diabetic coma waking up with the administration of insulin and glucose, but pernicious anaemia, as the name suggests, was a debilitating, distressing, and ultimately fatal affliction. Like insulin, however, the rationale for the therapy was based within the laboratory, in feeding experiments with dogs. The solution, eating large quantities of raw liver, was not exactly what patients might have chosen, but most thought it was better than the consequences of their disease.

These and other laboratory innovations – blood typing making transfusions safe, various vaccines, increased understanding of the nature of viruses – kept scientific medicine in the public domain. The take-off occurred in the years surrounding World War II, producing ultimately the big science that we still have. The sulpha drugs, for instance, were effective against several common bacteria: one consequence was a rapid decline in women's mortality from puerperal fever (the infection all too frequently following childbirth). These were developed just before the war (the Nazis refused to let their discoverer, Gerhard Domagk (1895–1964), go to Stockholm to collect his Nobel Prize), and the war itself put paid to the international patent system, so sulpha drugs could be manufactured outside of Germany. During the early years of the war, these drugs were much used; by its end, they had been overtaken by penicillin.

Penicillin is probably the wonder-drug of all time. Its story adds to the appeal, discovered in 1928 serendipitously by Alexander Fleming (1881–1955), through a mould on an uncovered Petri dish, but more or less neglected for a decade (there were a few isolated attempts to employ it therapeutically). With the outbreak of World War II, the Oxford professor of pathology Howard Florey

(1898–1968) and his team were charged with looking for new therapeutic agents against bacterial infections. Penicillin was among the substances they chose, and using makeshift equipment in wartime conditions, they isolated enough of the precious mould to show that it was indeed dramatically effective. Their first patient, an Oxford policeman with a staphylococcus infection following a rose-thorn puncture wound, improved, but there was not enough penicillin to achieve a cure, despite recovering it from his urine and readministering it. He died.

During the war, Florey and a colleague went to the United States, where pharmaceutical manufacturing was less disrupted. Florey had old-fashioned beliefs about the openness of scientific research, so failed to pay attention to the patent arrangements. American pharmaceutical manufacturers were much shrewder, and by the last two years of the war were manufacturing large quantities, and making large sums of money. At first, reserved essentially for military use (it was effective against many bacterial infections, including syphilis and gonorrhoea, as well as some contaminants of war wounds and bacterial pneumonias), penicillin was in general civilian use shortly after the war ended, in 1945.

The penicillin story is a thoroughly modern one. Highly profitable, it needed industrial modes of production and distribution. It was very effective against many common scourges, became cheap, saved many lives, and greatly increased the prestige of the laboratory and of modern medicine more generally. It was a miracle drug, even if miracles don't last forever. Penicillin was given indiscriminately, in doses that were not correct, for conditions that were not appropriate, and in courses that were not completed. It began to lose its effectiveness, as penicillin-resistant bacteria emerged. In the early days, this seemed only a minor problem, since other forms of penicillin were manufactured, and other antibiotics came on the market, including streptomycin, effective against tuberculosis, the age-old chronic bacterial killer. Streptomycin was developed in the United States, and when a small supply reached Britain just after the war, Austin Bradford Hill (soon to turn his attention to lung cancer) turned limited availability to good effect, designing a proper 'double-blind' controlled trial, in which neither the participating doctors nor the patients knew which therapy was being tested. In this way, the bias of expectation could be removed. The results demonstrated the therapeutic effectiveness of streptomycin. Hill's experimental design has become the gold standard for evaluating new therapies.

Streptomycin, penicillin, and the other antibiotics ushered in a golden age, when new effective drugs and vaccines seemed to be the inevitable result of pharmaceutical and biomedical research. Cortisone appeared in the late 1940s, and was accompanied by films showing severely crippled victims of rheumatoid arthritis getting out of their beds and walking. New drugs promised to control those cancers that were not within the reach of increasingly sophisticated surgery or radiotherapy. Antipsychotics dramatically reduced the symptoms of schizophrenia, severe depression, and the other afflictions of patients who had spent their lives in psychiatric asylums. Victims of encephalitis lethargica, an epidemic of the 1920s, who had been in a coma for decades, woke up in the late 1950s after being administered dopamine, a drug recently introduced for Parkinson's disease (the response was short-lived if dramatic). By the early 1960s, community psychiatry was the buzz word, as psychiatric patients were to be treated as outpatients, with the belief that they would be able to live more-or-less normal lives if they simply took their medicines. For people with mild depression or anxiety, Librium and Valium came on the market. Medicine seemed truly to have, or shortly to have, a pill for every ill.

Before the 1940s, most medical research in the United States was supported by private foundations and charities, of which the cancer, tuberculosis, and polio charities took centre-stage. Franklin D. Roosevelt's own polio kept this disease in the news.

In epidemic form, it became the major crippler of young people, with an average of 40,000 cases per year between 1951 and 1955. As a viral disease, it was not susceptible to antibiotics, and the consequence in those who survived the disease was often life-long disability. Although more prevalent in the United States than any other country, polio had a worldwide distribution (higher in the West than in poorer countries), and the epidemic in Copenhagen in 1952 was poignant, not only for its severity but for the acts of humanity it inspired. In order to keep the severely afflicted alive, tracheotomies and intermittent positive ventilation were used, with some 1,500 volunteers spending 165,000 hours ventilating polio victims by hand. Polio did not conform to the rich/poor divide: it is a disease of decent hygiene, children in countries without clean water acquiring the virus in infancy when it does not produce the lasting neuromuscular damage caused when older children and young adults are first exposed.

The viral aetiology of polio, and the fact that people who recovered never got the disease again, made a vaccine the most sensible strategy. The March of Dimes Foundation was wealthy, although grant applications were evaluated by standards that would be unacceptable today. Several vaccines were prepared in the 1940s, but only with the Salk and Sabin vaccines of the 1950s were large-scale immunization campaigns put into practice. Jonas Salk (1914–95) developed a killed-virus vaccine. Despite some serious glitches, the vaccine was effective, but it was soon superseded by the attenuated live-virus vaccine of Alfred Sabin (1906–93). Sabin's was administered orally, on a lump of sugar, which made it easy to distribute and popular with children. It had the advantage that the attenuated virus was then excreted in the faeces, and provided natural protection by the identical route (oral-faecal) through which the disease spreads. Like smallpox, polio is a modern success story and the disease's worldwide eradication has almost been achieved. The polio story is full of strong personalities, and no small amount of duplicitous behaviour, but the result was a desirable one.

Its success encouraged more medical research, and the vast industrial-scientific establishment we still have was created. The largest medical research organization in the world, the National Institutes of Health (NIH), in Bethesda, Maryland, was one beneficiary. From the 1950s, the American government began to be a major player in medical research, with ever larger laboratories and multi-authored scientific papers the norm. Whatever parameter one measures, basic medical research has increased dramatically over the past few decades. So have improvements in healthcare, at least in the West. Doctors in the early 21st century can diagnose and manage disease even better than they could in the 1970s. Asthma, cancer, peptic ulcer, cardiovascular disease, and many others are less likely to be sentences of invalidism and death than they were only a generation ago. The changing age profile means that chronic disease is more prominent, and the translation of medical research into clinical practice has meant that many of the gains of modern medicine relate to care, not cure. The promises of health improvements through sequencing the human genome or stem cell research are so far largely unrealized. As scientific capability rises, so do expectations, and many patients no longer have patience, having been promised so much.

Modern medicine: the reality of the new

It is perception as much as reality that dictates modern attitudes to medicine and what it can, and cannot, do. The thalidomide disaster was a turning point. It seemed an excellent drug in the late 1950s, a wonderful prevention of morning sickness in early pregnancy. It was hastily marketed and not adequately tested. A sharp-eyed official in the United States prevented its being released there, but thousands of women in more than 40 countries took the drug during pregnancy before the relationship between the drug and birth abnormalities in the limbs of their babies became clear. Although the episode ultimately did result in tightening up safety standards on new medicaments, it dented public confidence in the pharmaceutical industry. No subsequent

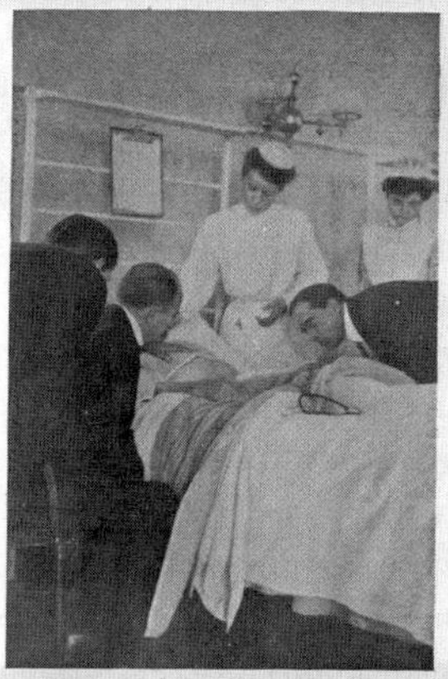

Inspection

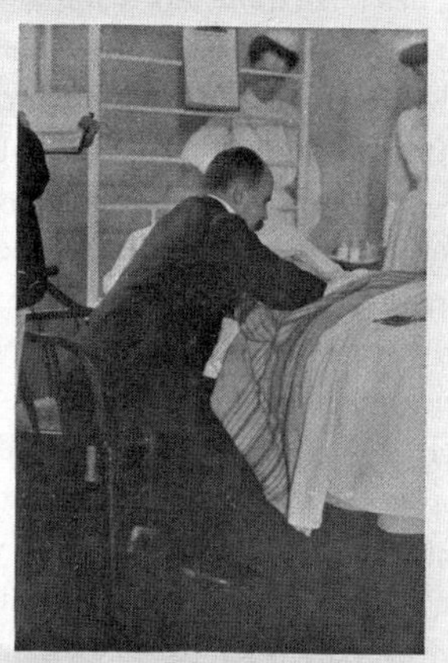

Palpation

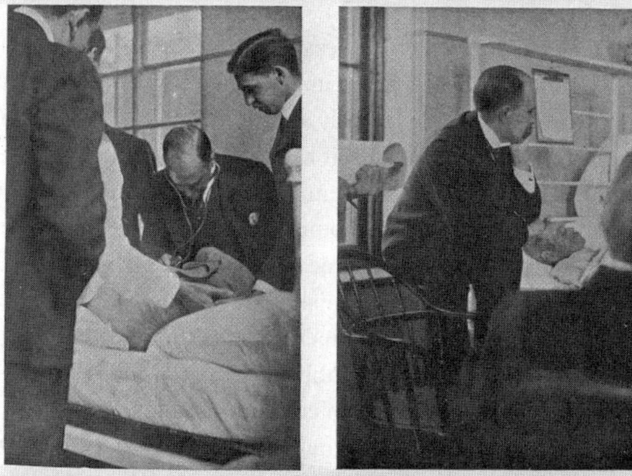

Auscultation

Contemplation

28. The studious physician at the bedside: Sir William Osler, one of the most admired physicians of all time, does his stuff in diagnosing and thinking about what he has learned. Bedside manner with modern intent

drug has been quite so obviously deleterious, even if several have been hastily withdrawn after side effects have emerged. The modern pharmaceutical industry has been of a piece with other multinational corporations. Small firms get swallowed up in larger ones, and contemporary budgets for advertising and sales are larger than those for research and development. Direct advertising of prescription-only drugs in the United States has introduced a new, disturbing element in the industry, and 'add-on' medicines, where small changes are made to an existing drug, occupy too much of the industry's time. Research tends to follow common disorders of the West, with lucrative potentials, instead of major diseases of the poorer countries, where there is great need but little chance of yielding vast profits. A long-term chronic disease, in which patients must take their medications for years, or even for the rest of their lives, is the ideal goal for a new drug.

HIV (AIDS) provides an object lesson on the status of modern market-driven healthcare. From its emergence in a particularly virulent form in the 1980s, largely among gay men and injecting drug users in the United States, it has become a symbol of the power and the problems of contemporary healthcare. Because it first manifested itself in a rich country, biomedical research was marshalled quickly, although some religious leaders insisted that the disease was simply God's punishment for homosexuality and other forms of sin. President Ronald Reagan took his time uttering the acronym AIDS in public and the Catholic Church refuses to countenance the use of condoms as a means of preventing the spread of this sexually transmitted disease. AIDS still carries the heavy burden of stigma.

If those at risk thought the official response was muted, this should be compared with traditional Western lethargy about diseases of poor countries that pose no threat to the rich ones. A quarter of a century later, the lapse between the earliest cases of Kaposi's sarcoma, then a rare form of cancer, and the appearance of compromised immune systems among previously healthy young adults, on the one hand, and the identification of the causative organism, in 1984, on the other, seems fairly short. That two groups, one in the United States and one in France, almost simultaneously identified the responsible retrovirus, and each claimed the spoils, is another sign of the times, when the big prizes in science are keenly contested.

HIV was initially known somewhat condescendingly as the disease of the 3 H's – homosexuals, heroin-users, and Haitians. The poor in Haiti were identified as an early vulnerable group, but they were soon joined by the African poor, and it is in Africa and other developing countries that the starkest issues and the most serious social and economic consequences of AIDS are found. In the West, the disease has quickly changed from an acute to a chronic one, although one still with a serious mortality rate. Antiviral treatments, available since the 1990s, slow the progress of the disease, but they remain expensive and have side effects. Good nursing care and the timely treatment of infections as they occur are also important in increasing quality of life and decreasing morbidity and mortality. Like so many diseases caused by micro-organisms, however, problems of drug resistance have come to the fore, and the HIV-positive tag is a grim one.

In some parts of Africa, AIDS is a disease commonly transmitted by heterosexual intercourse, and the incidence of individuals who are HIV-positive, as well as those suffering from the full-blown syndrome, is overwhelming. Treatment is expensive and in any case requires a healthcare infrastructure that is simply missing in most of the continent. Along with malaria and tuberculosis, AIDS has dominated the international health scene for the past couple of decades. All three diseases have strains that resist conventional chemical treatment and their knock-on effects in terms of morbidity and mortality in young adults are huge. Disease has further increased the differential between the rich and the poor and, despite the substantial contribution of the Gates Foundation and other international agencies, promises to do so in the immediate future.

AIDS has been called a social disease for which its sufferers looked to medical science for a solution. Science and medical practice based on it are among the most significant achievements of Western culture. We need them, but medical science alone cannot solve the problems of human beings. We no longer live in a world where the idea of inevitable progress carries much conviction.

References

Chapter 1

The quotations from the Hippocratic works 'On the Sacred Disease' and 'Aphorisms' are taken from Francis Adams (ed.), *The Genuine Works of Hippocrates*, 2 vols (London: The Sydenham Society, 1849). Shakespeare's question about the seat of fancy comes from *The Merchant of Venice*, Act 3.

Chapter 2

Sydenham's famous comment about the constancy of symptoms in different persons suffering from the same disease was made in his *Medical Observations*. I have used R. G. Latham (ed.), *The Works of Thomas Sydenham*, 2 vols (London: The Sydenham Society, 1848).

Chapter 3

Antoine Fourcroy's summary of the basis of Parisian medical education is quoted in Erwin Ackerknecht, *Medicine at the Paris Hospital, 1794–1848* (Baltimore: Johns Hopkins University Press, 1967); Bichat's ringing injunction also is quoted in Ackerknecht's monograph. The phrase 'gateways to death' as a description of bad hospitals originated with the physician and man of letters John Aikin (1747–1822), now better known as a writer than a physician. Francis

Bacon's phrase 'Footsteps of diseases' comes from his *Advancement of Learning*, originally published in 1605.

Chapter 4

Edward VII's stirring directive, said of tuberculosis, is quoted in Thomas Dormandy, *The White Death: A History of Tuberculosis* (London: Hambledon Press, 1999), with the note that Edward was cribbing from William Withering, the physician who introduced digitalis into clinical medicine in 1785. Mr Gradgrind's insistence on 'Facts' is a recurring trope in Charles Dickens's *Hard Times*, first published in 1854.

Chapter 5

Robert Hooke used the word 'cell' in his *Micrographia* (1665). Löffler's summary of the steps we know as 'Koch's Postulates' is quoted in Thomas D. Brock, *Robert Koch: A Life in Medicine and Bacteriology* (Madison, Wisconsin: Science Tech Publishers, 1988).

Chapter 6

William Wordsworth's memorable phrase first appeared in his poem 'The Tables Turned', published in 1798. Ivan Illich elaborated his notion of 'iatrogenesis' in several works, most centrally in *Medical Nemesis: The Expropriation of Health* (London: Calder and Boyars, 1975). C. P. Snow's lecture on what he called *The Two Cultures* was published by Cambridge University Press in 1959.

Further reading

General

W. F. Bynum and Helen Bynum (eds), *Dictionary of Medical Biography*, 5 vols (Westport, Connecticut, and London: Greenwood Press, 2007). Biographies of major medical figures from all over the world who have contributed to clinical medicine, plus introductory essays on the major medical traditions.

W. F. Bynum and Roy Porter (eds), *Companion Encyclopedia of the History of Medicine*, 2 vols (London: Routledge, 1993). A collection of essays covering the whole of the field.

W. F. Bynum, Anne Hardy, Stephen Jacyna, Christopher Lawrence, and E. M. (Tilli) Tansey, *The Western Medical Tradition, 1800–2000* (Cambridge: Cambridge University Press, 2006). A general survey of Western medicine during the past two centuries.

Lawrence I. Conrad, Michael Neve, Vivian Nutton, Roy Porter, and Andrew Wear, *The Western Medical Tradition, 800BC–AD1800* (Cambridge: Cambridge University Press, 1995). A general survey of the history of the Western medical tradition up to 1800.

Jacylyn Duffin, *History of Medicine: A Scandalously Short Introduction* (Toronto: University of Toronto Press, 1999). An excellent introduction, with good coverage of modern North American developments.

Stephen Lock, John M. Last, and George Dunea (eds), *The Oxford Illustrated Companion to Medicine* (Oxford: Oxford University Press, 2001). Arranged alphabetically, most of the articles have generous historical content.

John Pickstone, *Ways of Knowing: A New History of Science, Technology and Medicine* (Manchester: Manchester University Press, 2000). A stimulating introduction to these fields by a leading expert.

Roy Porter, *The Greatest Benefit to Mankind: A Medical History of Humanity from Antiquity to the Present* (London: HarperCollins Publishers, 1999). A widely admired, always readable survey.

Andrew Wear (ed.), *Medicine in Society: Historical Essays* (Cambridge: Cambridge University Press, 1992). An excellent collection of wide-ranging essays, especially written for teaching purposes.

David Weatherall, *Science and the Quiet Art: Medical Research and Patient Care* (Oxford: Oxford University Press, 1995). Historically sensitive study by an outstanding clinician and medical scientist.

Chapter 1: Medicine at the bedside

Noga Arokha, *Passions and Tempers: A History of the Humours* (New York: HarperCollins Publishers, 2007). A full history of the continuing influence of the doctrine of the humours within medicine and science.

M. D. Grmek, *Diseases in the Ancient Greek World* (Baltimore: Johns Hopkins University Press, 1989). An authoritative account of the evidence for the range of diseases prevalent in classical antiquity, using both written and material sources.

Helen King, *Hippocrates' Woman: Reading the Female Body in Ancient Greece* (London: Routledge, 1998). A stimulating account of women's diseases in ancient medical writings.

G. E. R. Lloyd (ed.), *Hippocratic Writings* (Harmondsworth: Penguin, 1978). A very useful selection of the Hippocratic writings with a fine introduction.

Vivian Nutton, *Ancient Medicine* (London: Routledge, 2004). A full and well-written survey by a leading scholar.

Owsei Temkin, *Galenism: Rise and Decline of a Medical Philosophy* (Ithaca: Cornell University Press, 1973). An account of Galen's continuing influence for more than a millennium after his death.

Chapter 2: Medicine in the library

Laurence Brockliss and Colin Jones, *The Medical World of Early Modern France* (Oxford: Clarendon Press, 1997). A monumental account of four centuries of medical life in France.

W. F. Bynum and Roy Porter (eds), *William Hunter and the Eighteenth-Century Medical World* (Cambridge: Cambridge University Press, 1895). A wide-ranging collection of essays on Enlightenment medicine and anatomy.

Peter Pormann and Emilie Savage-Smith, *Medieval Islamic Medicine* (Edinburgh: Edinburgh University Press, 2007). An up-to-date summary of a complex subject.

Roy Porter, *Quacks: Fakers and Charlatans in English Medicine* (Stroud, Gloucestershire: Tempus Publishing, 2000). An entertaining volume, rich in anecdote but also developing Porter's notion of the continuing importance of the medical marketplace.

Carole Rawcliffe, *Medicine and Society in Later Medieval England* (Stroud, Gloucestershire: A. Sutton, 1995). An accessible and wide-ranging survey.

Guenter B. Risse, *Hospital Life in Enlightenment Scotland: Care and Teaching in the Royal Infirmary of Edinburgh* (Cambridge: Cambridge University Press, 1986). An outstanding study of clinical medicine and medical education on the eve of the French Revolution.

Nancy G. Siraisi, *Medieval and Early Renaissance Medicine* (Chicago: Chicago University Press, 1990). An excellent introduction to the medicine of the period.

Chapter 3: Medicine in the hospital

Erwin H. Ackerknecht, *Medicine at the Paris Hospital, 1794–1848* (Baltimore: Johns Hopkins University Press, 1967). The classic study of the French school in the early 19th century.

W. F. Bynum, *Science and the Practice of Medicine in the Nineteenth Century* (Cambridge: Cambridge University Press, 1994). A general account of the increasing role of science within clinical medicine.

Jacylyn Duffin, *To See with a Better Eye: A Life of R. T. H. Laennec* (Princeton: Princeton University Press, 1998). A fine biography of the inventor of the stethoscope.

Michel Foucault, *The Birth of the Clinic: An Archaeology of Medical Perception*, tr. A. M. Sheridan Smith (London: Tavistock, 1973). One of the most accessible books of this influential thinker, in which he develops his ideas about power within medicine, focusing on the French clinical school.

Caroline Hannaway and Ann La Berge (eds), *Constructing Paris Medicine* (Amsterdam: Rodopi, 1998). A good series of essays by leading scholars, evaluating the French school.

Russell Maulitz, *Morbid Appearances: The Anatomy of Pathology in the Early Nineteenth Century* (Cambridge: Cambridge University Press, 1987). A stimulating study of the fortunes of pathology during its period of dominance within clinical medicine.

Guenter B. Risse, *Mending Bodies, Saving Souls: A History of Hospitals* (Oxford: Oxford University Press, 1999). An exceptionally elegant and thoughtful study of the hospital throughout history. Risse dissects the French hospitals of the early 19th century, discussed in Chapter 6.

Andrew Scull, *The Most Solitary of Afflictions: Madness and Society in Britain, 1700–1900* (New Haven and London: Yale University Press, 1993). Although focusing on Britain, Scull's powerful account highlights many common features of psychiatry and insanity throughout Europe and North America during this period.

Chapter 4: Medicine in the community

John Duffy, *The Sanitarians: A History of American Public Health* (Urbana, Ill.: University of Illinois Press, 1990). A sound account of the public health movement in the United States.

Christopher Hamlin, *Public Health and Social Justice in the Age of Chadwick: Britain, 1800–1854* (Cambridge: Cambridge University Press, 1998). An important study of the relationship between poverty and disease.

Daniel Kevles, *In the Name of Eugenics: Genetics and the Uses of Human Heredity* (Harmondsworth: Penguin, 1986). Still the best general account of the eugenics movement.

Ann La Berge, *Mission and Method: The Early Nineteenth-Century French Public Health Movement* (Cambridge: Cambridge University Press, 1992). An excellent synthesis of the French movement.

Thomas McKeown, *The Role of Medicine: Dream, Mirage or Nemesis?* (Oxford: Blackwell, 1979). The most pungent statement of McKeown's vision of medicine and its history.

Dorothy Porter, *Health, Civilization and the State: A History of Public Health from Ancient to Modern Times* (London: Routledge, 1999). A good synthesis of a vast topic.

Dorothy Porter (ed.), *The History of Public Health and the Modern State* (Amsterdam: Rodopi, 1994). A fine collection of essays on many countries, by leading experts.

Chapter 5: Medicine in the laboratory

Erwin H. Ackerknecht, *Rudolf Virchow: Doctor, Statesman, Anthropologist* (Madison: University of Wisconsin Press, 1953). This old biography is still an excellent introduction to the many facets of Virchow's career.

Claude Bernard, *An Introduction to the Study of Experimental Medicine*, tr. Henry Copley Green (New York: Dover Publications, 1957). Originally published in 1865, Bernard's classic monograph is still well worth reading.

William Coleman and Frederic Lawrence Holmes (eds), *The Investigative Enterprise: Experimental Physiology in Nineteenth-Century Medicine* (Berkeley: University of California Press, 1988). An outstanding collection of essays on experimental physiology and its relevance for medical practice.

Patrice Debré, *Louis Pasteur*, tr. Elborg Forster (Baltimore: Johns Hopkins University Press, 1998). A full biography of Pasteur, sympathetic but not uncritical.

Henry Harris, *The Birth of the Cell* (New Haven and London: Yale University Press, 1998). A good introduction to 19th-century microscopy.

Owen H. Wangensteen and Sarah D. Wangensteen, *The Rise of Surgery: From Empiric Craft to Scientific Discipline* (Folkestone, Kent: Dawson, 1978). Old-fashioned and in the heroic mode, but wonderfully cosmopolitan and accurate in its details.

Michael Worboys, *Spreading Germs: Disease Theories and Medical Practice in Britain, 1865–1900* (Cambridge: Cambridge University Press, 2000). A subtle investigation of the impact of bacteriology and germs theories on British medicine.

Chapter 6: Medicine in the modern world

Michael Bliss, *The Discovery of Insulin* (Edinburgh: Harris, 1983). A balanced account of this famous episode in the history of medicine.

Thomas Neville Bonner, *Becoming a Physician: Medical Education in Great Britain, France, Germany and the United States, 1750–1945* (Oxford and New York: Oxford University Press, 1995). A fine comparative study, with many resonances for earlier chapters of this Introduction as well.

Roger Cooter and John Pickstone (eds), *Medicine in the Twentieth Century* (Amsterdam: Harwood Academic Publishers, 2000). A large collection of essays on many aspects of medicine in the last century.

John Farley, *The International Health Division of the Rockefeller Foundation: The Russell Years, 1920–1934* (Cambridge: Cambridge University Press, 1995). An excellent introduction to the important dimension of international health, and the Americanization of the world.

Joel Howell, *Technology in the Hospital: Transforming Patient Care in the Early Twentieth Century* (Baltimore: Johns Hopkins University Press, 1995). A fine monograph on how medical science and technology influenced what doctors did in the hospital.

James Le Fanu, *The Rise and Fall of Modern Medicine* (London: Little, Brown and Co., 1999). A perceptive account of 20th-century medicine by a shrewd general practitioner and medical journalist.

Harry Marks, *The Progress of Experiment: Science and Therapeutic Reform in the United States, 1900–1990* (Cambridge: Cambridge University Press, 1997). An excellent introduction to the clinical trial, and much else besides.

Rosemary Stevens, *In Sickness and in Wealth: American Hospitals in the Twentieth Century* (New York: Basic Books, 1989). A full analysis of the economic and medical dimensions of American hospitals.

Index

Q

R

S

T

U

V

W

X

DRUGS
A Very Short Introduction
Leslie Iverson

The twentieth century saw a remarkable upsurge of research on drugs, with major advances in the treatment of bacterial and viral infections, heart disease, stomach ulcers, cancer, and mental illnesses. These, along with the introduction of the oral contraceptive, have altered all of our lives. There has also been an increase in the recreational use and abuse of drugs in the Western world. This book explains what drugs are, how they work, and how medicines are developed and tested. It also discusses current ideas about why some drugs are addictive, and whether drug laws need reform.

'extremely interesting and capable . . . although called a very short introduction, it contains a wealth of information for the interested layman and is exemplary in its accuracy.'

Malcolm Lader, King's College, London

'a slim but assured and wise volume on drugs. [It] takes up many controversial positions . . . with an air of authority that commands respect. It is difficult to think of a better overview of the field for anyone new to it.'

David Healy, University of Wales College of Medicine

www.oup.co.uk/isbn.0-19-285431-3